HIIT

The 20-Minute Dream Body with High Intensity Interval Training

2nd Edition

By John Powers

Copyright© 2014 by John Powers - All rights reserved.

Copyright: No part of this publication may be reproduced without written permission from the author, except by a reviewer who may quote brief passages or reproduce illustrations in a review with appropriate credits; nor may any part of this book be reproduced, stored in a retrieval system, or transmitted in any form or by any means – electronic, mechanical, photocopying, recording, or other - without prior written permission of the copyright holder.

The trademarks are used without any consent, and the publication of the trademark is without permission or backing by the trademark owner. All trademarks and brands within this book are for clarifying purposes only and are owned by the owners themselves.

Disclaimer: The information in this book is not to be used as professional medical advice and is not meant to treat or diagnose medical problems. The information presented should be used in combination with guidance from a competent professional person.

The information within the book "HIIT – The 20-Minute Dream Body with High Intensity Interval Training" is intended as reference materials only and not as substitute for professional advice. Information contained herein is intended to give you the tools to make informed decisions about your body physical level and ability to perform exercises. Every reasonable effort has been made to ensure that the material in this book is true, correct, complete and appropriate at the time of writing.

The Author and Publisher has strived to be as accurate and complete as possible in the creation of this book, notwithstanding the fact that he does not warrant or represent at any time that the contents within are accurate due to the rapidly changing nature of the subject and the Internet (third party website links). Nevertheless the Author and Publisher assume no liability or responsibility for any omission or error, for damage or injury to you or other persons arising from the use of this material. Reliance upon information contained in this material is solely at the reader's own risk.

Any perceived slights of specific persons, peoples, or organizations are unintentional. Like any other sport, HIIT poses some inherent risk. The Author and Publisher advice readers to take full responsibility for their safety and know their limits. It is also recommended that you consult with a qualified healthcare professional before beginning any training on the subject. Before practicing the skills described in this book, be sure that your equipment is well maintained, and do not take risks beyond your level of experience, aptitude, training and comfort level.

First Printing, 2014 - Printed in the United States of America

2nd Edition - Revised and Expanded.

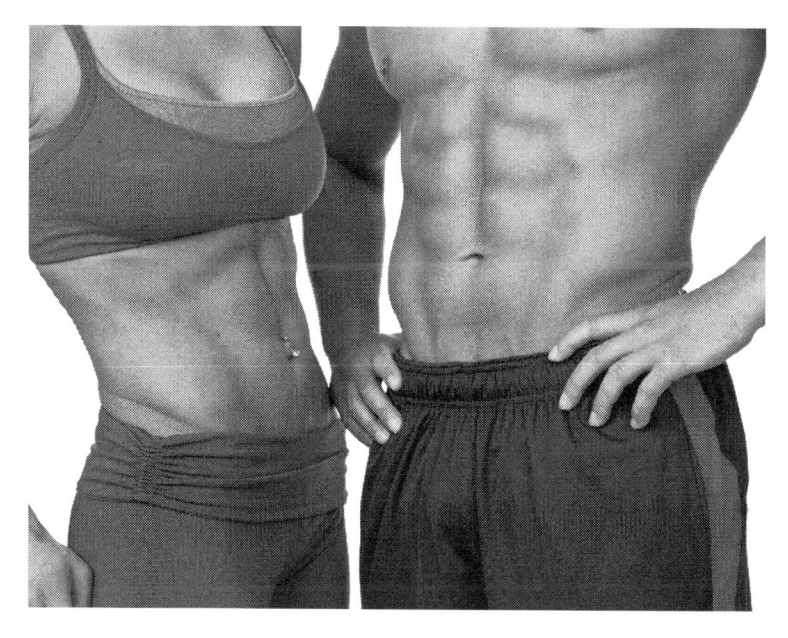

"High-intensity interval training is one of the hottest fitness trends in 2014"

- American College of Sports Medicine

TABLE OF CONTENTS

Why a Revised Edition	1
Introduction	3
Chapter 1 – What is HIIT?	5
Background	7
Who Can Perform HIIT?	8
Benefits of HIIT	9
HIIT Workout Programs	11
How HIIT Compares to Other Workout Programs	13
Concerns with HIIT Programs	15
Chapter 2 – The Science Behind HIIT	17
Energy and the Body's Use of Oxygen	19
Sleep – The Surprising Connection	21
Aerobic Aspects of HIIT	22
Anaerobic Aspects of HIIT	23
Overtraining Syndrome	25
It Comes Down to the Fuel	28
Chapter 3 – HIIT and Nutrition	29

Understanding the Fueling Process	30
It's All About Carbohydrates…	32
…But Not Just Carbohydrates	34
Your Diet and HIIT	36
Don't Neglect Proper Hydration	40
A Word About Toxins	41
Chapter 4 – HIIT and Weight Loss	**43**
The Body Becomes a Fat Burning Machine	45
HIIT Makes the Entire Body Work Hard	47
Lose Weight While You Rest	48
What About Calories?	49
When and What to Eat?	52
Targeting Those 'Problem Areas'	54
Chapter 5 – HIIT and Cardio	**55**
Make Any Cardio Activity a HIIT Cardio Workout	56
Sample Cardio Workouts	59
Chapter 6 – HIIT and Cross-Training	**63**
Cross Training Workouts	65
Scheduling Cross Training Sessions	71
Choosing HIIT Workout Activities	72

Sample HIIT Workout Progression	73
Chapter 7 – HIIT and Endurance	75
What Is Improved Endurance?	76
How HIIT Benefits Overall Endurance	77
HIIT Programs for Different Types of Endurance	79
How Much is Too Much?	81
Chapter 8 – HIIT and Weight Lifting	83
Incorporating HIIT into a Weight Lifting Regimen	84
How HIIT Cardio Boosts Weight Training Success	86
A Word About Nutritional Supplements	87
Chapter 9 – Sample Exercises and How to Perform Them	89
Exercise Options for HIIT Workouts	99
Chapter 10 - FAQ	105
Conclusion	111
About the Author	113

WHY A REVISED EDITION

Firstly, I would like to thank everyone who took their time to review this book and send some constructive feedback. I really appreciate that.

After considering comments by several readers, it became evident that some clarifications needed to be made to the text. In an effort to make the book better and easier to follow, several sections were expanded and some explanations added to address areas that were not as clear as they could have been. Also, several questions and answers were added into Chapter 10 – FAQ in response to reader suggestions. On top of that, a bonus 7-minute HIIT Workout Program has been added for those who can't spare 20 minutes a day to become fit.

This book is designed to help everyone learn about and begin a HIIT program regardless of current levels of physical ability or function. There was no intent to exclude beginners or those with limited physical skills – just the recommendation of developing some cardiovascular endurance before attempting the rigorous program that HIIT is designed to provide. As with any new physical pursuit or for anyone with medical concerns, discuss the program with a health care professional for the optimal results and to prevent injury.

Creating a HIIT program is an individual process designed to accommodate the interests and abilities of the participants. Variety over time is crucial as your body gets used to the activities and timing you choose and recovery is also an important aspect of any plan for participants at all levels. HIIT is great as a complete exercise plan and even better as an addition to specific workout protocols for sports, weight lifting or running.

Enjoy reading this book, follow the suggestions and you will be surprised at the speed with which you see results!

JOHN POWERS

INTRODUCTION

Do you wish you could lose weight, have a great, ripped physique and keep up with your activities with greater stamina? If you are like most people, you certainly do! Today, these goals are actually much easier to achieve than most people think.

Unlike many exercise programs, **High Intensity Interval Training *(HIIT)* allows** more people **to see measurable improvement in** as few as **14 days with just 3 sessions of 20 minute workouts each week**. That means super fat burning potential, muscle sculpting and much better endurance.

Make your personal transformation a reality by reading and adopting the information in the next 10 chapters into your lifestyle. **This book will give you easy to follow exercise plans and interval timing tips** along **with diet and recovery advice**.

Let's take a quick look at what this is all about. Many different exercise trends have come and gone over the years but HIIT has been growing increasingly in popularity. This workout involves brief intervals of extremely high intensity activity alternated with recovery periods that are repeated for a total of only 20 to 30 minutes of exercise. It sounds easy – especially the short length of the workout – but it is really quite demanding. And that is why it works so well!

HIIT has been around in a variety of forms for many years already but is becoming more prominent among a wide range of athletes and fitness enthusiasts. As early as the 1930s, runners trained using timed bursts of increased speed incorporated in their usual routine to build overall speed and stamina. During the 1940s, a similar method was adopted by the US Marine Corps Office Candidates School to improve the results of their training cycle.

Today, there is plenty of advice regarding the best HIIT programs. DVDs, YouTube and written material offer advice, suggestions and encouragement that make it easy for just about anyone to realize what they never thought possible in terms of personal fitness and appearance.

This book is designed to provide you with:

- an introduction to HIIT

- the science behind the success of HIIT

- a range of useable tips and techniques for beginners and even accomplished athletes

- the application of HIIT to a number of different types of workout routines and disciplines

As with any weight loss effort, diet is an important consideration so *you will also find information about appropriate nutrition and hydration*. You will be surprised to find out that 'diet' doesn't mean eating only salad!

Although proven professional advices have been provided throughout this book, the diet and workout plans are suggestions that should be considered carefully and modified for individual needs. It is important for everyone to consult with their health practitioner before beginning any exercise program.

So turn the page and **find out how you can beat all the excuses and get down to work creating the body you have always wished for!**

CHAPTER 1 – WHAT IS HIIT?

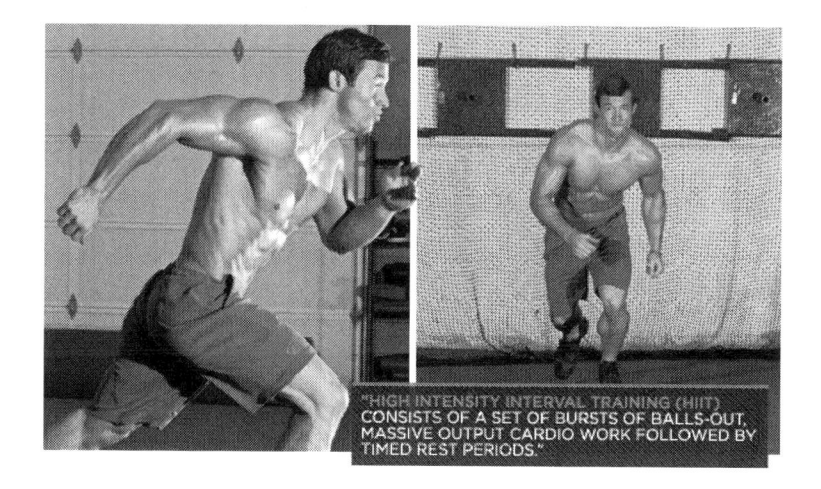

"HIGH INTENSITY INTERVAL TRAINING (HIIT) CONSISTS OF A SET OF BURSTS OF BALLS-OUT, MASSIVE OUTPUT CARDIO WORK FOLLOWED BY TIMED REST PERIODS."

Simply defined, **HIIT** or **High Intensity Interval Training** is a specific type of *athletic workouts that alternate quick, intense bursts of exercise followed by short recovery periods*. HIIT is not a particular program but any activity or set of activities that can be adapted for intensity and duration.

The real key to HIIT is that the intense phase of the exercise is done at nearly 100% effort and the recovery phase is movement at 60% to 70% of maximum effort, still within the fat burning range.

The **basic features setting HIIT apart** from other workout routines include:

- HIIT uses all major muscle groups
- Is performed only 3 times per week
- Alternates cardio and full-body power moves
- Takes only 20 to 30 minutes
- Maximizes weight loss without loss of muscle mass

Background

Alternating short periods of intense activity with regular activity was the idea of a Swedish running coach in 1937. This plan, *Fartlek* - which means 'speed play' in Swedish, trains and enhances both the aerobic and anaerobic energy systems of the body. Runners were able to significantly improve their speed and stamina after adopting this training method.

During the 1940s and 1950s, the practice of interval training began with the addition of 'wind sprints' or 'alternates' to traditional workout sessions. It was supported by research into 'work tolerance' but was not standardized with the specific identification of work and rest intervals. It was discovered that an athlete suffers exhaustion and lactic acid build-up when performing different activities even though the work level was the same as the workout that was 'easy'. In other words, for overall strength and stamina**, each muscle group needs to be addressed in training** and not just the muscles involved in a particular activity.

Moving ahead to the 1970s, it became fairly common practice for athletes to add another discipline to their workout routines and the concept of ***cross training*** was born. NFL football teams added ballet training to improve dexterity and balance and other types of athletes added weight training to complement stamina and address more areas of their bodies than their sport-specific training developed. Effective cross training focuses on the most functional elements of a variety of disciplines in combination to promote overall endurance and strength of all muscle groups.

Together, the **concepts of interval training and cross training have combined** and evolved **into** the discipline of **High Intensity Interval Training**. HIIT takes advantage of a wide variety of activities and training methods for the best overall body shaping, fat burning, conditioning and endurance.

Who Can Perform HIIT?

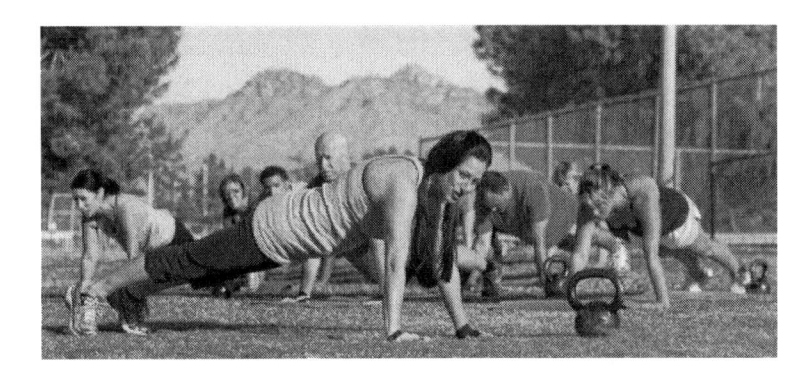

Part of the appeal of HIIT is the fact that virtually anyone interested in an intense, focused workout plan can participate in these activities. Younger or older, world-class athlete or the 'average Joe', HIIT can be modified to suit everyone's needs and abilities. Of course, as with any new program, it is best to consult with your health care provider to ensure that the rigors of HIIT are within your physical ability.

Obviously, beginners and experienced fitness enthusiasts will train at different levels. For each person and even the same person on different days, the workout takes as much as can be given since it does not follow a plan for a set number of reps or certain milestones. **Everyone puts in as close to 100% intensity as possible** – whatever that means to each and every individual at any particular point in time.

Another tremendous advantage of **HIIT workouts** is that they are quick and **can be done anytime and anywhere** – no need for a gym, special equipment or a personal trainer if that is what you choose.

Benefits of HIIT

High Intensity Interval Training involves coordinated effort of all the body's muscle groups and systems to bring about the *most rapid weight loss* (if that is the intention) while *improving strength, endurance and overall physical ability*. The intensity of participation determines the effectiveness of the approach. Simply raising the heart rate is not enough – HIIT requires true all-out effort that should leave you exhausted at the end of the workout.

When done properly, **HIIT offers many benefits** over other, more traditional types of cardio workouts and other exercise programs.

- **Increases metabolism:** The intensity of the HIIT workout boosts metabolism for up to 48 hours after completing a full routine. Production of Human Growth Hormone (HGH) is stimulated which helps to increase caloric burn, especially fat, as well as slows the aging process.

- **Increases 'afterburn effect':** HIIT sessions increase the body's need for oxygen during recovery – 'Excess Post-Exercise Oxygen Consumption' (EPOC) – which helps burn more fat and calories than even-paced workouts of a long duration or traditional aerobic activity.

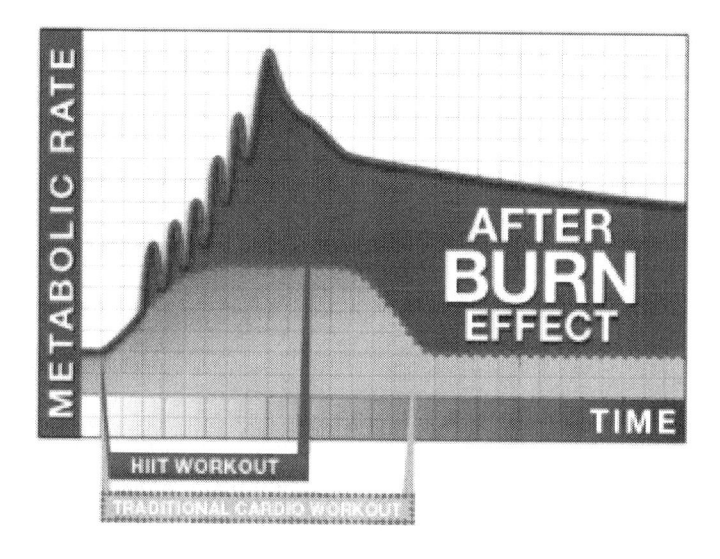

- **Improves aerobic capacity** in about 2 weeks as much as 6 to 8 weeks of traditional endurance training.

- **Improves heart health**: HIIT gets you to the anaerobic zone quicker and more efficiently.

- **Reduces blood-sugar levels** in Type 2 diabetics in as little as 2 weeks.

- **Eliminates exercise boredom**: Short intervals and the incorporation of many different types of activities keep HIIT workouts fresh and motivating.

- **Challenging**: With short-term goals, it is easy to see progress and feel success.

- **Quick**: HIIT workouts should not last more than 20 or 30 minutes so they can fit into anyone's schedule.

- **Convenient**: HIIT can be performed anywhere with a minimum of equipment or just your own body weight so it is great for at home, on the road or in the gym.

HIIT Workout Programs

Although HIIT workouts can be devised with any activity utilizing timed intervals of intense work and recovery, there are several programs with specific guidelines.

The Fartlek Method is essentially interval training and can be adapted to virtually any activity although it was originally designed to improve the performance of runners. The main point of this method is to vary the intensity of portions of your workout, alternating slow and moderate paced movement with maximum intensity bursts. Speed and intensity can be adjusted along with actual duration of activity and rest periods that imitate competitive action.

Fartlek works both the aerobic and anaerobic systems and reduces the boredom of steady-paced activity such as running, swimming or biking. Timing can be an issue, especially when you want to do multiple sets so a coach, partner or pre-recorded play-list are ways to stay on track.

The Tabata HIIT workout is named for a Japanese speed skating team coach who studied the effects of the head coach's protocol on the athletes. The process of training in explosive bursts with short rest periods was improving not only strength but endurance as well. The results were published in *'Medicine and Science in Sports and Exercise'* in 1996 and describe what is now known as the Tabata Protocol.

Ideally, the athlete performs at 170% of VO2max in alternating intervals of 20 seconds work and 10 seconds of recovery for 8 to 10 sets. A full Tabata workout actually lasts only 4 to 5 minutes (after a 5 minute warm up) due to the extreme exertion required and should be done only 2 to 4 times per week.

The 'Gibala Regimen', also known as 'The Little Method' has two workout programs suitable for both athletes and beginners. Studied at McMaster University, Canada, this method involves 3 minutes of warm up, and intervals of 60 seconds of intense activity (95% of VO2 max) followed by 75 seconds of rest with 8 to 12 reps. The 'lighter' approach uses the same warm up but intervals of 60 seconds of work (80-95% of VO2 max) with 60 seconds of recovery and a cool down period. This method can be performed 3 times per week.

The '10-20-30' program, devised by Danish researchers whose study was published in 2012, has also proven to have tremendous results regarding overall endurance training, reducing blood pressure and cholesterol in athletes and casual participants. This protocol involves a 5 minute warm up and intervals of 30 seconds of low intensity, 20 seconds of medium intensity and 10 seconds of high intensity repeated 5 times, followed by 2 minutes of rest and repeated for a total of 4 or 5 sets, all of which are completed within 20 to 30 minutes.

How HIIT Compares to Other Workout Programs

Essentially, **HIIT combines the concepts of interval and cross training** for an overall, full-body workout at an intense level for maximum calorie burn and long-term residual effects. To compare HIIT to either type of workout – just intervals or just cross training - is to look at only half the picture. Additionally, any activity such as running or weight lifting that targets just one area or basic set of motions is incomplete in terms of overall fitness.

Based on the research conducted regarding **the most efficient physical workouts for strength, stamina, metabolic enhancement and most efficient weight loss**, a number of programs have been created that incorporate this new exercise philosophy.

Several examples that can be used as part of a HIIT plan include:

CrossFit is a program that was developed by combining different types of fitness training to achieve the most significant overall fitness results without over-emphasizing any one particular area. CrossFit's broad focus applies to the improvement of agility, balance, cardio-vascular endurance, muscle strength, power, speed and stamina. It is a gym-based program that utilizes a wide range of equipment and the input of trainers.

MetCon3 at *Senergy Fitness* is another intense workout that combines strength training and anaerobic conditioning drills. This is a circuit-style timed workout performed in a gym with a combination of 4 to 10 exercises repeated in multiple rounds with little rest. The goal is to complete as many reps as possible within the time allowed while maintaining good form and remaining near your anaerobic threshold.

Turbo Fire (HIIT) and the Insanity Workout provides high-energy cardio exercise without the use of exercise machines or other pieces of equipment so it can be enjoyed in a class or at home. While Turbo Fire incorporates HIIT philosophy, it is not a complete HIIT program. It focuses on cardio kickboxing while the Insanity Workout involves calisthenics, cardio, plyometrics and sports drills.

Zumba and dance fitness classes enjoy a great deal of popularity because they are fun and can be done in a class or at home with the help of a video or DVD. The drawback in terms of overall fitness is that these activities are primarily cardio and don't address muscle strength or different muscle groups.

Concerns with HIIT Programs

The obvious concern regarding High Intensity Interval Training is, of course, the **intensity**. You must be in relatively good health and at a respectable fitness level before tackling the demands of HIIT.

That is not to say, however, that relative beginners can't benefit from HIIT activities. It is important to know and accept your limits but there are so many options for workout disciplines, you can find those that create the least stress or discomfort. For example, a stationary bike or swimming can be much easier for many people than running. Using resistance bands instead of weights presents another option that better suits some preferences and ability levels.

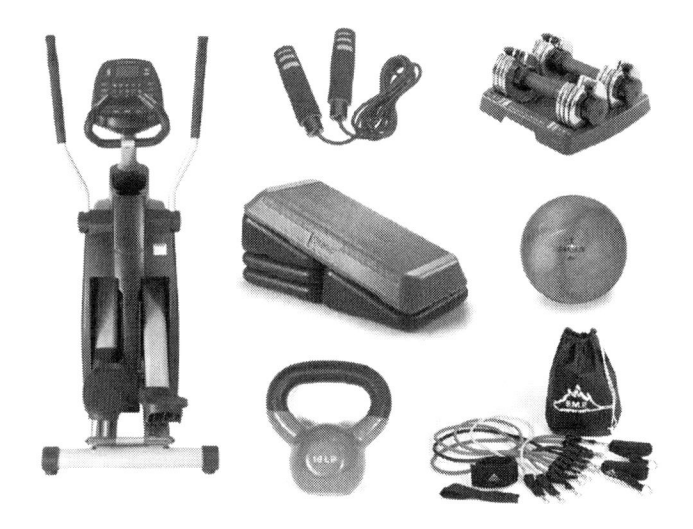

Intensity is measured differently for every individual and there are plenty of HIIT plans that allow you to get used to the demands of the program at your own pace. The beauty of HIIT is that is incorporates intense and moderate activity in a simple ratio so if you can't sustain the hard work for 1 minute, aim for just 30 seconds and set your 'recovery' period accordingly. (Intervals and timing will be discussed in later chapters.).

Another area for concern with HIIT workouts is **nutrition**. It is important to understand not only your body's overall caloric needs but also the sources of those calories in order to properly fuel your muscles for the demands you will place on them. HIIT creates much more complex physiological reactions within the body than traditional exercise routines.

As with any exercise program, you should consult with your health care professional before you begin to ensure safe, injury-free success.

CHAPTER 2 – THE SCIENCE BEHIND HIIT

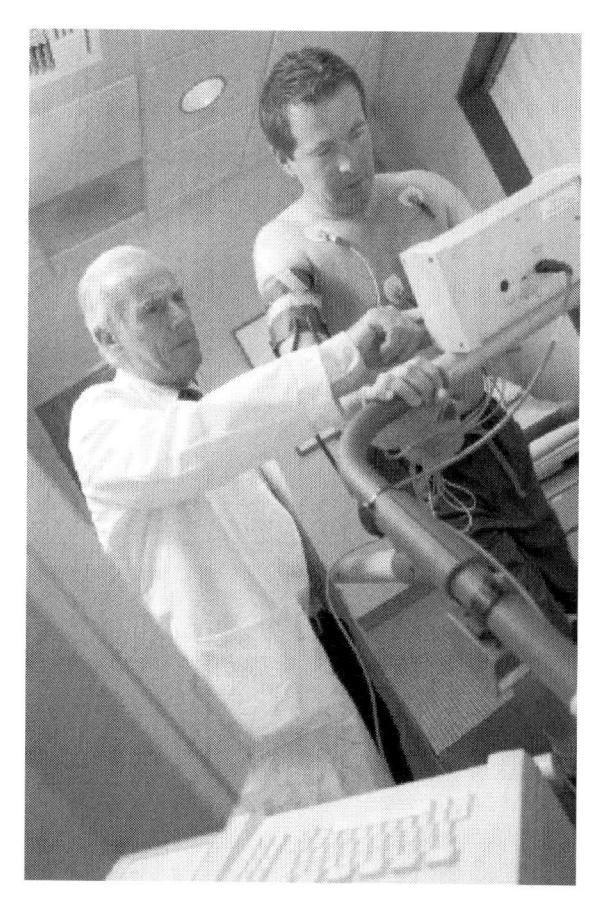

Sports and fitness physiology has received quite a bit of attention over the past several decades as professionals aim for greater strength, better performance and enhanced endurance. Research methods have also significantly improved so that even changes at the cellular level can be observed, measured and compared in relation to different types of exercise and the nutrition that supports the body.

In terms of the benefits of HIIT, there are several key concepts that explain why you look and feel better after completing your sessions. **The effectiveness of HIIT** is the result of the combination of physiological and neurological processes that last for extended periods of time after the workout, continuing to affect the body much longer than other traditional forms of exercise.

Energy and the Body's Use of Oxygen

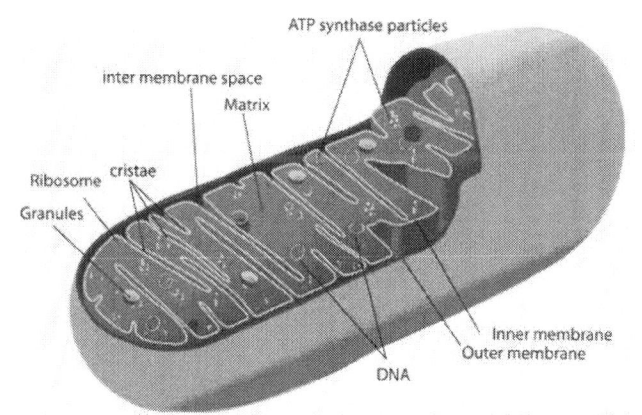

Diagram of a mitochondrion with labels: ATP synthase particles, inter membrane space, Matrix, Ribosome, cristae, Granules, Inner membrane, Outer membrane, DNA.

Mitochondria help to maintain proper concentration of calcium ions within the various compartments of the cell.

Mitochondria stores calcium.

The major function of the mitochondria is to produce energy.

Mitochondria helps in the formation of blood components and hormones such as testosterone and estrogen.

Mitochondria in the liver helps to detoxify ammonia.

Production of heat is another function of mitochondria.

Mitochondria helps in the regulation of membrane potential, cell proliferation and cell metabolism.

Mitochondria cause apoptosis or programmed cell death.

Mitochondria helps in the the biosynthesis of heme and steroids.

The human body is an amazing machine that is well-calibrated to perform thousands of chemical reactions automatically. There is constantly the production of fuel in the form of **ATP** (*adenosine triphosphate*) that is stored in the cells, ready to be released to synthesize enzymes, sugars and hormones as well as other substances for the purpose of cellular growth, reproduction and tissue repair.

This production of ATP is an aspect of metabolism called **'catabolism'** or the series of chemical reactions that break down complex compounds into their constituent elements such as amino acids from proteins, and simple carbohydrates from complex carbohydrates.

During this on-going process, the body also makes demands for energy to perform activities. This side of metabolism is called *anabolism* and the ratio between the two, anabolism and catabolism, determines the relative weight of the body. If there is little call for energy, the body then stores glycogen in the form of fat in the event of a future need. In other words, the body becomes fat.

Oxygenation of the cells takes place in the tiny components called ***mitochondria***. This aerobic respiration is responsible for creating the majority of our body's ATP. When the number and density of the mitochondria are increased through high intensity exercise, they are better able to transform lipids (fat-like substances such as cholesterol) into ATP and spare the glycogen stored in the body.

In simpler terms, improving the function of your mitochondria is like putting a bigger engine in a car. This allows you to perform longer at a higher intensity and with less accumulation of lactic acid and other cellular wastes including free radicals. In fact, it has been shown that high intensity training with periods of exercise and rest leads to increased enzyme content in the mitochondria which affect a variety of metabolic pathways.

When you engage in any activity, the body only has so much energy available whether you are a world class athlete or a couch potato. The challenge to the cells to provide adequate energy for any increased work load causes the mitochondria to respond by growing or adding new ones. This is especially important for overweight individuals and those who suffer from type 2 diabetes since the regulation of blood sugar is a large part of this process.

Sleep – The Surprising Connection

As a well-functioning machine, the body can handle a variety of changes and stresses but a **factor that has a tremendous impact on the overall efficiency of all internal systems is sleep**. Unsatisfying or inadequate sleep affects the *neuroendocrine* levels that control appetite and can lead to overeating for several reasons.

Not only are the signals alerting the brain of hunger and fullness affected, the fat cells themselves are less sensitive to insulin which can result in the altering of insulin resistance and increasing a person's risk for developing type 2 diabetes and obesity. Food choices also changed to carbohydrate-rich items, especially in the evening. Overall, growth hormones and thyroid stimulating hormone (*TSH*) are altered and there is an elevation of low grade inflammation which points to a relatively significant metabolic disruption. (*The Metabolic Consequences of Sleep Deprivation* Kristen L. Knutson, Karine Spiegel, Plamen Penev, Eve Van Cauter).

Additionally but not surprisingly, being tired leaves a person less likely to be interested in or even able to exercise depending on the actual degree of fatigue and the compounded effects of poor dietary choices.

Aerobic Aspects of HIIT

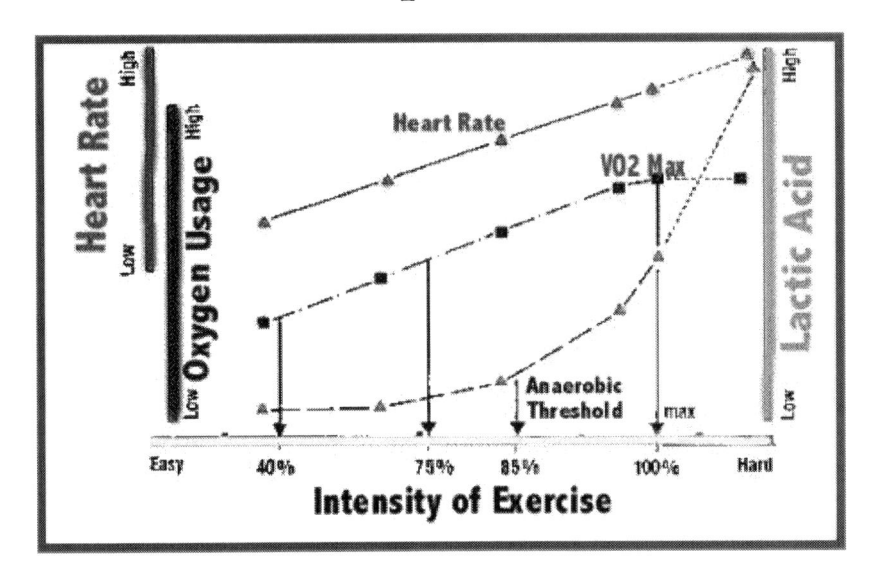

Most people have heard the term *'aerobics'* and probably associate it with cardio-type exercises. During aerobic activity, the mitochondria are consuming oxygen and catabolically converting glycogen and fat to fuel- ATP. When HIIT is performed, the body is pushed to its limits so that mitochondrial biogenesis (creation of new mitochondria) is promoted and there is an overall improvement in their efficiency and ability to burn even more fat and remove greater levels of carbon dioxide and other cellular waste products.

With the increase in oxygen intake during HIIT activities and the resulting boost to the mitochondria, other chemical reactions in the body are enhanced. Human Growth Hormone (HGH) which is responsible for burning fat, building muscles and strengthening bones is produced at greater levels. This is an excellent way to help combat the effects of aging!

Catecholamine levels also rise significantly and this directly stimulates the mobilization of fat cells for the conversion into useable energy.

Aerobic, cardio and endurance exercises such as jogging, running (at a mild pace), swimming and biking tend to 'fire' slow twitch (Type I) muscle fibers which happen to contain the most mitochondria. The result is a stronger heart and lungs, more efficient fat burning, improved mood and lowered risk of diabetes.

Anaerobic Aspects of HIIT

Energy Used By Muscles

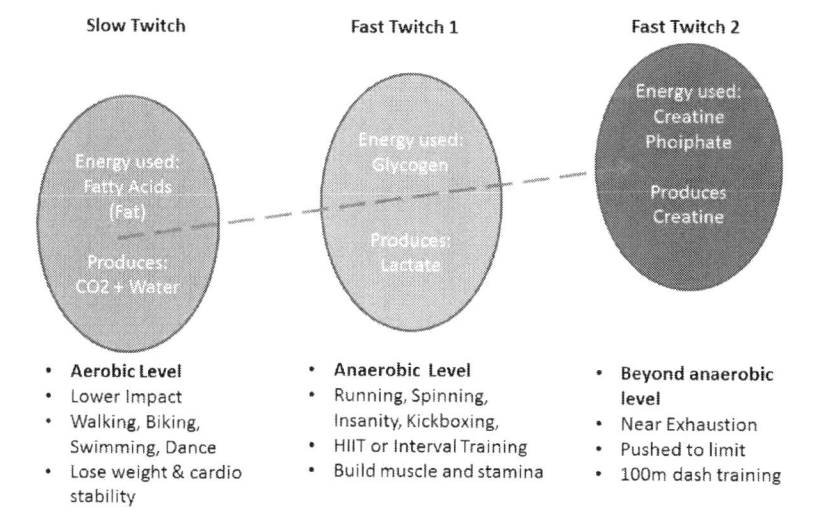

Slow Twitch
- Energy used: Fatty Acids (Fat)
- Produces: CO2 + Water

- **Aerobic Level**
- Lower Impact
- Walking, Biking, Swimming, Dance
- Lose weight & cardio stability

Fast Twitch 1
- Energy used: Glycogen
- Produces: Lactate

- **Anaerobic Level**
- Running, Spinning, Insanity, Kickboxing,
- HIIT or Interval Training
- Build muscle and stamina

Fast Twitch 2
- Energy used: Creatine Phoiphate
- Produces Creatine

- **Beyond anaerobic level**
- Near Exhaustion
- Pushed to limit
- 100m dash training

Anaerobic activity is **performed in the absence of oxygen**. What this means is that 'fast twitch' (Type II A & B) muscles that depend solely on glycogen that is stored in the muscles for fuel fire in intense, relatively short bursts.

Whereas aerobic activity can occur over a long period of time as in distance running or moderately riding a bike, anaerobic activity such as heavy weight lifting, interval training, jumping rope or any type of sprinting is of much shorter duration but much more intense.

The benefits of anaerobic exercise center around **building strength and muscle mass** as opposed to significant cardio-vascular improvements but it does also improve your VO2max and endurance. The significance of oxygen consumption during anaerobic exercise is not in the performance of the activity itself but for better cellular response in the recovery period afterwards.

During intense exercise, lactic acid, which is a waste product of anaerobic energy production, can build up in the muscles and become quite uncomfortable. As your training advances and you continue to push your limits, your body will be better able to tolerate this build up and then remove it more efficiently so the onset of fatigue is delayed. In some cases, this 'buffering' of lactic acid and its effects can be improved by between 10 and 50%.

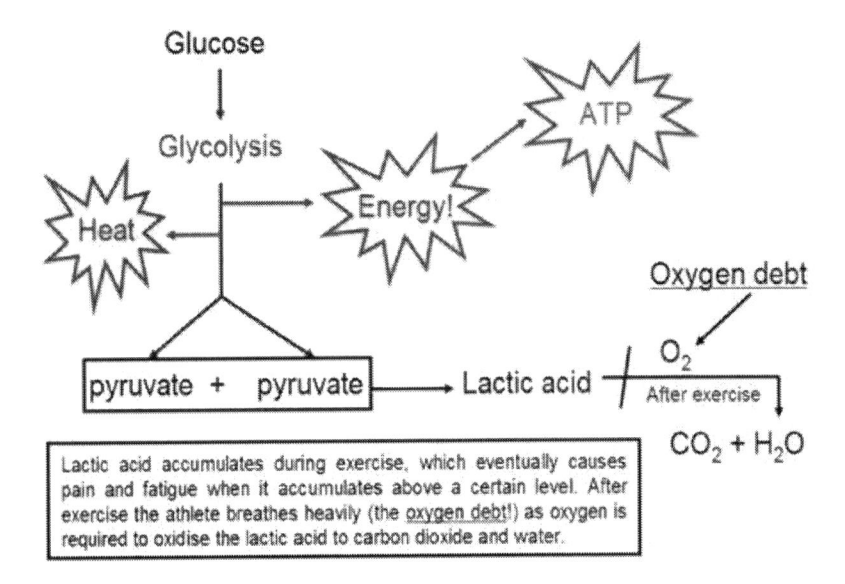

```
                    Glucose
                       |
                   Glycolysis                    ATP
        Heat  ←        |        →  Energy!   ↗
                       |                              Oxygen debt
                       ↓                              ↗
              ┌──────────────────┐              O₂
              │pyruvate + pyruvate│ → Lactic acid ─┤ After exercise
              └──────────────────┘              ↓
                                              CO₂ + H₂O
```

Lactic acid accumulates during exercise, which eventually causes pain and fatigue when it accumulates above a certain level. After exercise the athlete breathes heavily (the oxygen debt!) as oxygen is required to oxidise the lactic acid to carbon dioxide and water.

Due to the intense nature of anaerobic exercise in general but especially when performed along HIIT guidelines, it should not be performed by people who don't already have a good degree of fitness. Even with proper preparation, it is important to warm up with aerobic activity first. When incorporating anaerobic elements in a HIIT workout, the critical fact to remember is to rest appropriately between intervals to remove lactic acid and replenish the muscle's energy through oxygenation. Remember, muscle oxygenation takes longer than blood oxygenation or catching your breath and is crucial for the proper functioning of cellular activity.

Overtraining Syndrome

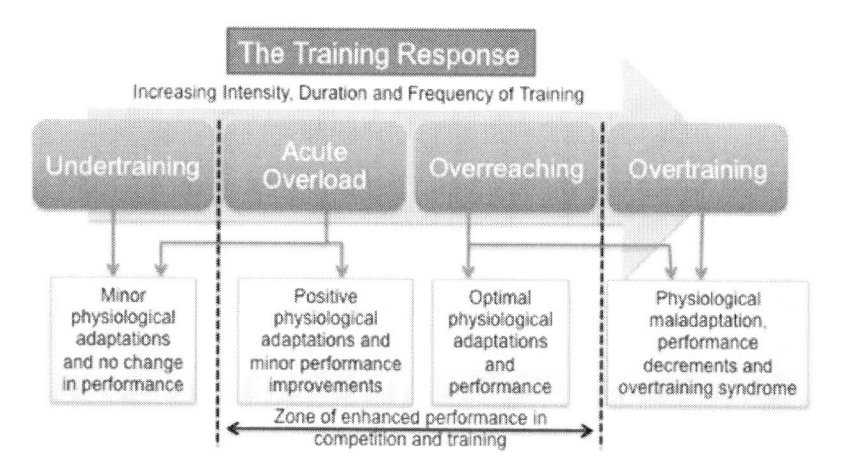

The Training Response
Increasing Intensity, Duration and Frequency of Training

Undertraining	Acute Overload	Overreaching	Overtraining
Minor physiological adaptations and no change in performance	Positive physiological adaptations and minor performance improvements	Optimal physiological adaptations and performance	Physiological maladaptation, performance decrements and overtraining syndrome

Zone of enhanced performance in competition and training

Have you ever reached a plateau in your training or wondered why you are losing ground instead of making improvements? The reason this occurs is usually what is called '*Overtraining Syndrome*'. What this means is that a higher volume, intensity or frequency in training, if not handled properly with appropriate lower intensity intervals and rest periods, can result in Central Nervous System (CNS) Fatigue.

Previously in this chapter, the concept of 'challenging' the mitochondria to grow and multiply was mentioned. Instead of using the term 'challenging', use the term 'stressing' and you have a more accurate picture of the physiological mechanism that encourages the body to adapt.

Stress, whether it is from an increased workout or a bad day at the office, **causes the production of the hormone *cortisol*** which raises blood pressure and blood sugar while lowering the body's immune and inflammatory responses. Too much cortisol can also lead to a decrease in muscle tissue and an increase in abdominal fat.

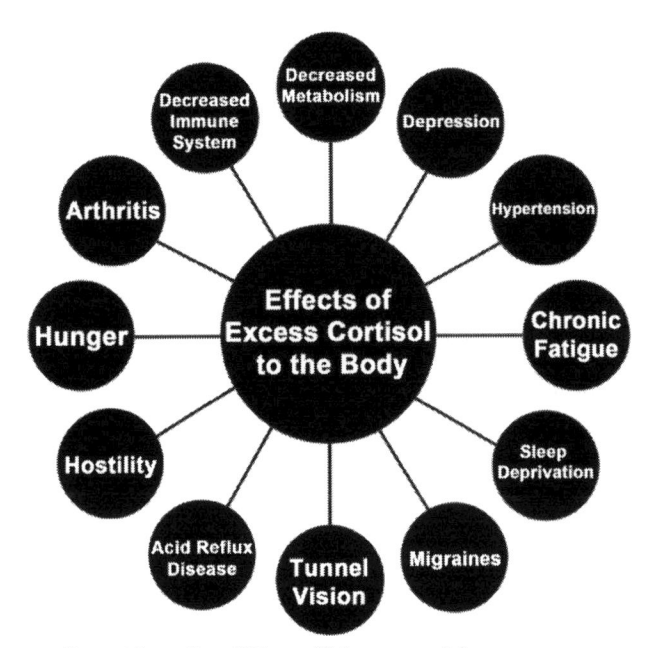

Effects of Excess Cortisol to the Body: Decreased Metabolism, Depression, Hypertension, Chronic Fatigue, Sleep Deprivation, Migraines, Tunnel Vision, Acid Reflux Disease, Hostility, Hunger, Arthritis, Decreased Immune System

Cortisol - The Stress Hormone

The only way to combat the effects of cortisol release is to properly engage the relaxation response. This means adequate rest breaks during HIIT activities and the limitation of these workouts to just several times a week. Maintaining proper hydration and diet are also key factors in reducing the risk of this type of fatigue. (Other stress-causing factors need to be addressed and removed from your life, but that is another issue entirely.)

There are numerous physical and mental *signals that point to overtraining*:

- Overall lack of energy

- Soreness in the legs along with other aches and pains

- Increased resting heart rate

- Headaches

- Sudden drop in performance and even loss of interest in the sport

- Increase in the number of immunity related problems - colds, sore throats and injuries

- Inability to sleep

- Decrease in appetite

- Compulsive need to exercise

- Mental slowness

- Moodiness

- Depression

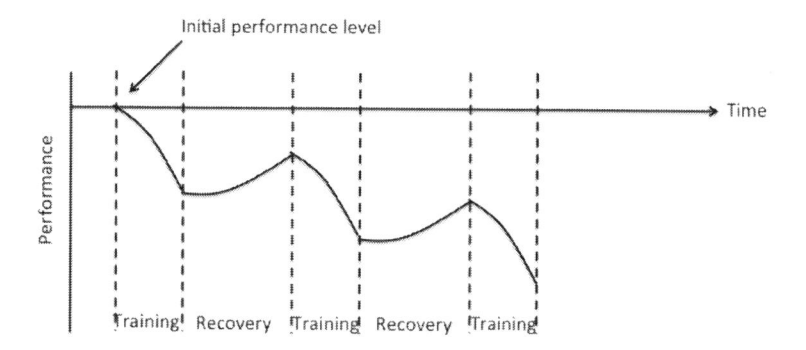

Model of overtraining: Training load followed by insufficient recovery results in decreased performance.

Homeostasis, or the inherent tendency of the body to maintain stability, is an amazing adaptive function. The brain sends these signals of stress and fatigue so that you realize that something is wrong and stop what you are doing before it leads to real injury. For that reason, it is crucial to listen to your body and not focus on a prescribed routine or to keep shooting for the 'high' of dopamine flooding your system.

It Comes Down to the Fuel

Now that you understand a little about how the body functions, it is time to consider what role nutrition plays in your ability to perform every-day activities as well as handle the significant demands created by HIIT workouts.

In the next chapter, you will discover the relationship between different sources of energy and the best foods to supply the unique requirements of intense activity.

CHAPTER 3 – HIIT AND NUTRITION

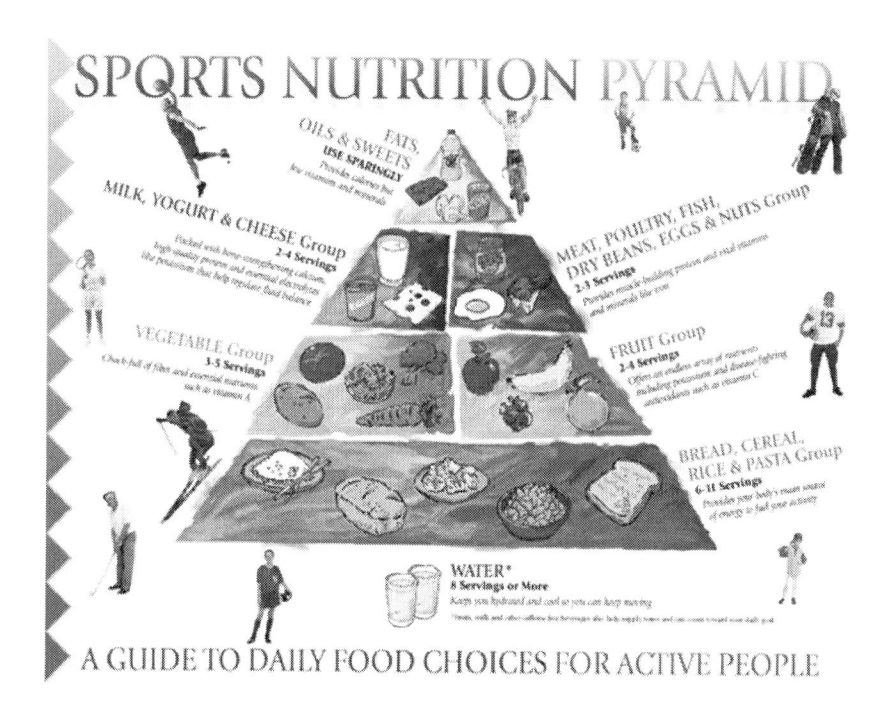

The body is a fantastic machine in which the proper nutrients play a key role for optimal functioning. A healthy, fit body requires the appropriate range of vitamins, minerals, proteins and carbohydrates from a variety of food sources to provide all the building blocks for high energy and good health.

Understanding the Fueling Process

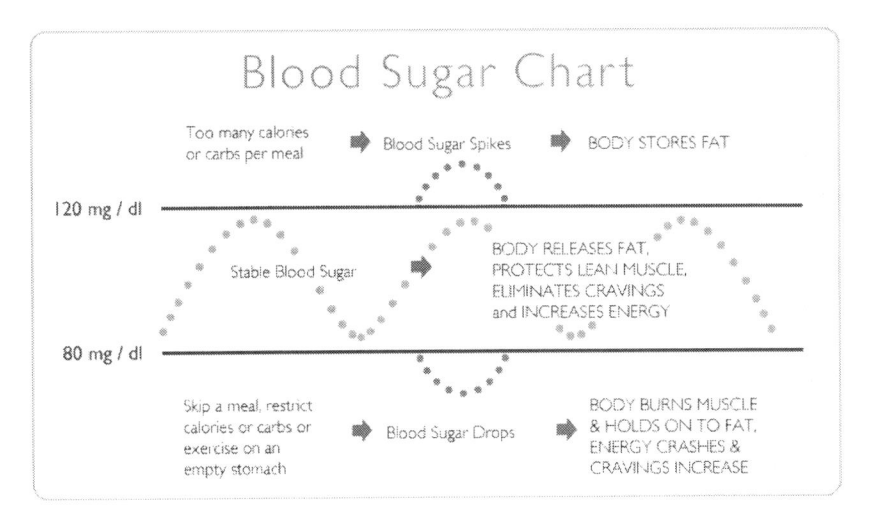

Blood Sugar Chart

- Too many calories or carbs per meal ➡ Blood Sugar Spikes ➡ BODY STORES FAT
- 120 mg / dl
- Stable Blood Sugar ➡ BODY RELEASES FAT, PROTECTS LEAN MUSCLE, ELIMINATES CRAVINGS and INCREASES ENERGY
- 80 mg / dl
- Skip a meal, restrict calories or carbs or exercise on an empty stomach ➡ Blood Sugar Drops ➡ BODY BURNS MUSCLE & HOLDS ON TO FAT, ENERGY CRASHES & CRAVINGS INCREASE

When you consider a diet, quite often the first thing you hear is to reduce or eliminate carbohydrates. While there is a certain degree of merit to that statement, it is a tremendous over-simplification that has a significant effect on your ability to exercise, especially the high endurance and intense activities of HIIT.

As a matter of fact, any 'drastic' dietary change such as overloading on protein or eating only fruits and vegetables results in tremendous challenges to the nutritional balance the body requires.

Misunderstandings regarding the nutritional requirements of the body and the need for the appropriate 'fuel' for the cells to function optimally are the primary reason many diets fail and can even result in gaining weight, particularly with the addition of an exercise program.

As we discussed in <u>Chapter 2: The Science Behind HIIT</u>, the body is an extremely complex machine that is constantly re-calibrating itself in an effort to maintain homeostasis. When you abruptly change one element of the body's routine, it has a ripple effect which in turn changes other functions and reactions.

To put it more clearly, let's continue with the machine analogy.

- If you use a cheaper or less well refined source of fuel, the engine will perform differently.

- If you were to change round parts to rectangles, the machine would not work as efficiently.

- If you take out some gears or relays, the remaining system has to work harder to get the same job done.

- If you expect the same machine to do the job of two, it will not handle the load.

Now let's apply that picture to the human body. Nutrition can come from candy bars or natural, raw foods and you can certainly tell where this is going! A candy bar may give you a quick jolt of energy but you can't live on that type of diet without disastrous consequences. The 'round parts and rectangles' are figurative representations for the nutritional building blocks required for proper cellular, and therefore, muscle function. If you don't provide the right elements or choose to use unnatural forms such as supplements in place of whole foods, the pieces don't mesh properly.

Taking out gears or relays and expecting a significant increase in output equate with simply not having enough of the right nutrients to perform the job of creating energy. The end result is working the body to the point of 'hitting the wall' or complete fatigue.

It's All About Carbohydrates...

Going back to the topic of carbohydrates, you can now see that removing them from the diet could present a problem. Here is the reason why: **carbohydrates are the source of the energy that fuels muscle function**.

The misunderstanding about carbohydrates comes from the fact that we think of 'carbs' as the elements in bread, pasta, cookies and such that pack on the fat. That is definitely true in a very broad sense but in strictly nutritional terms, *carbohydrates in the body* constitute the primary fuel supply that is broken down into smaller sugars that are used immediately for cellular energy or stored as glycogen in the muscles and liver or as fat in the body.

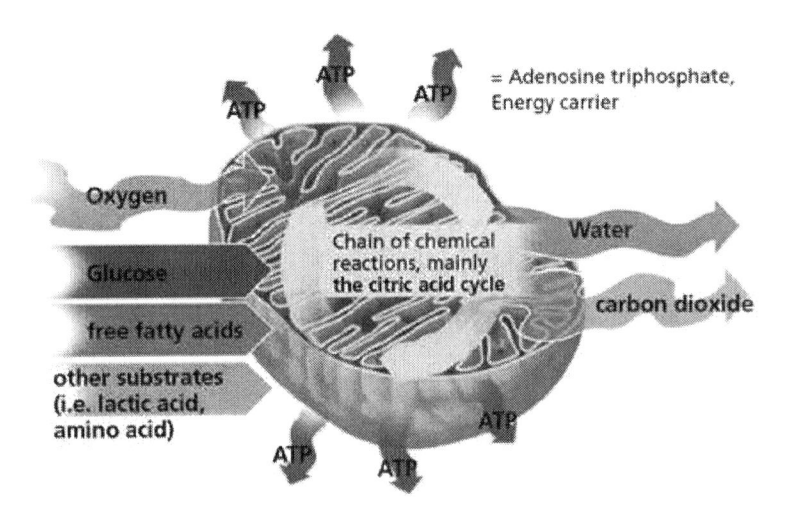

In cases of extreme carbohydrate deficiency, the body no longer has glycogen to use as fuel so it begins to metabolize its own protein. This leads to the breakdown of muscle, hair, bone and skin and forces the kidneys to work harder in order to eliminate the waste products associated with this type of protein synthesis.

Just to be clear about the *importance of dietary carbohydrates*, these complex chains not only provide the energy needed for cellular growth and function but also:

- Regulate blood sugar levels

- Provide nutrients for probiotics in the intestinal tract that promote proper digestion

- Aid in the absorption of calcium

- Assist in regulating blood pressure and controlling cholesterol levels

- Fuel the CNS (Central Nervous System) and the brain.

...But Not Just Carbohydrates

Back to the broad interpretation of what carbohydrates are! Any school student should be able to tell you about the daily recommended dietary requirements needed for good health. The 'Food Pyramid' and other graphic representations of what foods are needed for the body to work properly include proteins from fish, fowl, lean meats and nuts, vegetables and fruits, whole grains, dairy, healthy fats and oils and limited amounts of refined grains, potatoes, white rice (carbohydrates!) and only minimal amounts of other items such as salt, sugar and processed foods.

The body needs a variety of foods to supply the vast array of nutrients needed for optimal health and function. For people interested in regaining or maintaining their health, **adding protein, vitamins and minerals from natural sources and eliminating processed foods** are the most important steps toward promoting proper nutrition.

There is no ideal diet plan, however, because there are many factors that contribute to a person's food choices. The important thing to realize, though, is that there are many options (just look at the selections in any supermarket!) and common sense backed by some education should lead to making the best nutritional decisions. When trying to **'plan' a diet strategy**, there are **some ideas to keep in mind**:

- Pay more attention to the dietary choices you make

- Focus on the quality of the food you eat – that doesn't mean cost but amount of processing

- A broad range of selections helps to eliminate possible nutrient deficiencies

- Control the urge to eat – by eating better, you usually feel more satisfied and eat less

- Remain active – when you feel better and have more energy with a good diet, you are also more inclined to get involved with an increase in physical activity which in turn improves the body's ability to utilize the nutrients you provide more efficiently.

GLYCEMIC INDEX CHART
Low Glycemic (55 or Below)   High Glycemic (70 or Higher)

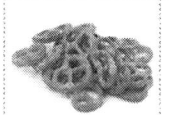

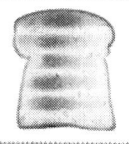

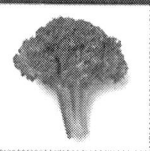

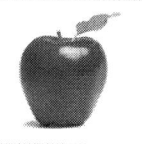

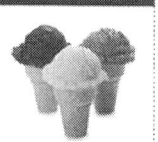

SNACKS	G.I.	STARCH	G.I.	VEGETABLES	G.I.	FRUITS	G.I.	DAIRY	G.I.
Pizza	33	Bagel, Plain	33	Broccoli	10	Cherries	22	Yogurt, Plain	14
Chocolate Bar	49	White Rice	38	Pepper	10	Apple	38	Yogurt, Low Fat	14
Pound Cake	54	White Spaghetti	38	Lettuce	10	Orange	43	Whole Milk	30
Popcorn	55	Sweet Potato	44	Mushrooms	10	Grapes	46	Soy Milk	31
Energy Bar	58	White Bread	49	Onions	10	Kiwi	52	Skim Milk	32
Soda	72	Brown Rice	55	Green Peas	48	Banana	56	Chocolate Milk	35
Doughnut	76	Pancakes	67	Carrots	49	Pineapple	66	Yogurt, Fruit	36
Jelly Beans	80	Wheat Bread	80	Beets	64	Watermelon	72	Custard	43
Pretzels	83	Baked Potato	85	Onions	75	Dates	103	Ice Cream	60

Glycemic Index values obtained from www.lowglycemicdiet.com, www.nutritiondata.com and www.diabetesnet.com

Your Diet and HIIT

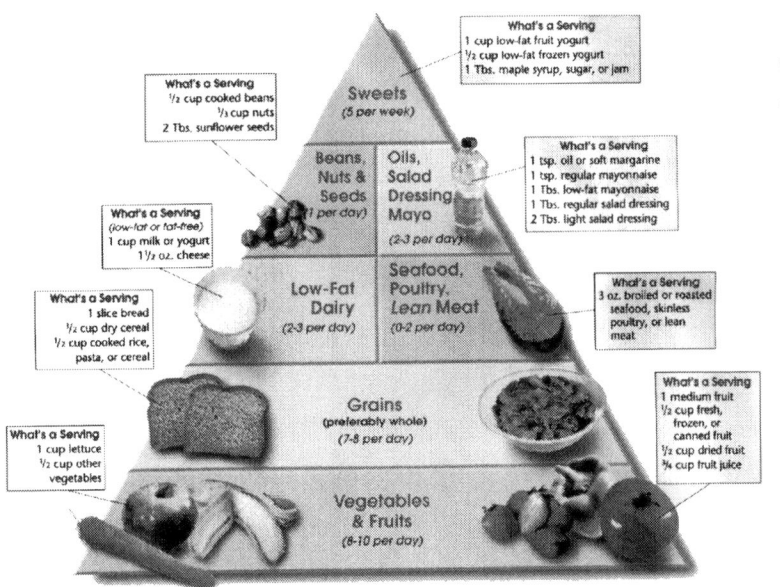

Food Pyramid:
- **Sweets** (5 per week) — What's a Serving: 1 cup low-fat fruit yogurt; ½ cup low-fat frozen yogurt; 1 Tbs. maple syrup, sugar, or jam
- **Beans, Nuts & Seeds** (1 per day) — What's a Serving: ½ cup cooked beans; ⅓ cup nuts; 2 Tbs. sunflower seeds
- **Oils, Salad Dressing, Mayo** (2-3 per day) — What's a Serving: 1 tsp. oil or soft margarine; 1 tsp. regular mayonnaise; 1 Tbs. low-fat mayonnaise; 1 Tbs. regular salad dressing; 2 Tbs. light salad dressing
- **Low-Fat Dairy** (2-3 per day) — What's a Serving: (low-fat or fat-free) 1 cup milk or yogurt; 1½ oz. cheese
- **Seafood, Poultry, Lean Meat** (0-2 per day) — What's a Serving: 3 oz. broiled or roasted seafood, skinless poultry, or lean meat
- **Grains** (preferably whole) (7-8 per day) — What's a Serving: 1 slice bread; ½ cup dry cereal; ½ cup cooked rice, pasta, or cereal
- **Vegetables & Fruits** (8-10 per day) — What's a Serving: 1 cup lettuce; ½ cup other vegetables / 1 medium fruit; ½ cup fresh, frozen, or canned fruit; ½ cup dried fruit; ¾ cup fruit juice

Note: Choose lower-salt foods from all categories.

When you decide to participate in HIIT workouts, just like you should have some degree of fitness, you should also start with a relatively healthy diet. If you live on pizza and beer, take a few weeks of eating a more well-rounded diet aiming for better nutritional choices.

Equally as important, if you are on a highly restricted carbohydrate diet, allow some time for your body to adjust to eating more quality carbohydrates to ensure an adequate glucose supply to provide enough energy to successfully complete a workout.

Some *additional dietary suggestions* include:

- Eat breakfast every day

- Boost **fruit and vegetable** intake to 7 **colorful servings** per day and include lemons or lemon juice

- Take 10 g of **fish oil** per day

- Select foods rich in **Omega-3 fat**

- Eat a small portion of a **lean protein** with every meal and snack

- Make smart carb choices at each meal (starches and other **low Glycemic Index carbs** are preferable to sugars and other high GI carbs)

- Drink **green tea** and avoid caffeine (since it is a diuretic and removes needed fluid from the body)

- Consume whole foods along with herbs and spices* to help to ease inflammation, promote detoxification, aid digestion and assist in recovery (*Anise, Basil, Burdock, Cilantro, Cinnamon, Cayenne, Cloves, Cumin, Garlic, Ginger, Ginseng, Licorice, Milk Thistle, Mint, Nutmeg, Oregano, Rosemary, Sage, Schizandra, Thyme, Turmeric)

Here's how *sample bodybuilder's meal plan* would look like:

Meal 1

1 Banana	140 cals	35g carbs	2g protein	1g fat
2 Eggs (boiled)	140 cals	2g carbs	12g protein	9g fat
.5c Oats	150 cals	27g carbs	5g protein	3g fat
1c 1% Milk	110 cals	13g carbs	8g protein	3g fat
Total =	540 cals	77g carbs	27g protein	16g fat

Meal 2

2 Whey Scoops	260 cals	6g carbs	52g protein	4g fat
1 Banana	140 cals	35g carbs	2g protein	1g fat
1 PB&J Sandwich	310 cals	34g carbs	12g protein	21g fat
Total =	710 cals	75g carbs	66g protein	26g fat

Meal 3

1 Can Tuna	100 cals	2g carbs	22g protein	2g fat
2 Slices Bread	90 cals	18g carbs	5g protein	1g fat
.5c Brown Rice	110 cals	21g carbs	3g protein	2g fat
Total =	300 cals	41g carbs	30g protein	5g fat

Meal 4

.5c Oats	150 cals	27g carbs	5g protein	3g fat
1 Banana	140 cals	35g carbs	2g protein	1g fat
1 Scoop Whey	130 cals	3g carbs	26g protein	2g fat
1c 1% Milk	110 cals	13g carbs	8g protein	3g fat
Peanut Butter 2TBL	180 cals	6g carbs	7g protein	16g fat
Total =	710 cals	84g carbs	48g protein	25g fat

Meal 5

1 Chicken breast	240 cals	0g carbs	44g protein	6g fat
1c Mixed Veggies	25 cals	4g carbs	1g protein	0g fat
.5c Brown Rice	110 cals	21g carbs	3g protein	2g fat
Total =	375 cals	25g carbs	48g protein	8g fat

Meal 6

.5c Cottage Cheese	120 cals	4g carbs	12g protein	6g fat
2 Eggs (boiled)	140 cals	2g carbs	12g protein	9g fat
Total =	260 cals	6g carbs	24g protein	15g fat

Daily Totals	2895 cals	308g carbs	243g protein	95g fat
Macros	646 grams	48% carbs	38% protein	15% fat

HIIT

And here's a *sample of weight loss meal plan*:

Meal	100-120lbs	120-160lbs	160-200lbs	200-240lbs	240-280lbs
Breakfast	6 egg whites Salsa 1 tbsp olive oil 1 banana	6 egg whites Salsa 1 tbsp olive oil 1 banana	6 egg whites Salsa 1 tbsp olive oil 1 banana 1 slice of whole grain bread	6 egg whites Salsa 1 tbsp olive oil 1 banana 1 slice of whole grain bread	6 egg whites Salsa 1 tbsp olive oil 1 banana 1 slice of whole grain bread
Mid-Morning	½ cup Greek Yogurt 2 tbsp flaxseeds	½ cup Greek Yogurt 1 cup blueberries 2 tbsp flaxseeds	½ cup Greek Yogurt 1 cup blueberries 2 tbsp flaxseeds	½ cup Greek Yogurt 1 cup blueberries 2 tbsp flaxseeds	½ cup Greek Yogurt 1 cup blueberries 1 cup strawberries 2 tbsp flaxseeds
Lunch	3 oz chicken breast 1 small whole wheat tortilla Sliced veggies 1 tbsp olive oil salad dressing	3 oz chicken breast 1 small whole wheat tortilla Sliced veggies 1 tbsp olive oil salad dressing	3 oz chicken breast 1 small whole wheat tortilla Sliced veggies 1 tbsp olive oil salad dressing 1 orange	6 oz chicken breast 1 small whole wheat tortilla Sliced veggies 1 tbsp olive oil salad dressing 1 orange	6 oz chicken breast 1 small whole wheat tortilla Sliced veggies 1 tbsp olive oil salad dressing 1 orange
Mid-Afternoon	1 scoop whey protein powder 10 almonds	1 scoop whey protein powder 1 apple 10 almonds	1 scoop whey protein powder 1 apple 10 almonds	1 scoop whey protein powder 1 apple 10 almonds	1 scoop whey protein powder 1 apple 1 banana 10 almonds
Dinner	3 oz lean steak 5 spears asparagus 1 tbsp olive oil 1 tbsp lemon juice	3 oz lean steak 5 spears asparagus 1 tbsp olive oil 1 tbsp lemon juice	6 oz lean steak 5 spears asparagus 1 small sweet potato 1 tbsp olive oil 1 tbsp lemon juice	6 oz lean steak 5 spears asparagus 1 small sweet potato 1 tbsp olive oil 1 tbsp lemon juice 1 cup strawberries	6 oz lean steak 5 spears asparagus 1 small sweet potato 1 tbsp olive oil 1 tbsp lemon juice 1 cup strawberries
Before Bed	½ cup low-fat cottage cheese 1 tbsp natural peanut butter	½ cup low-fat cottage cheese 1 tbsp natural peanut butter	½ cup low-fat cottage cheese 1 tbsp natural peanut butter	½ cup low-fat cottage cheese 1 tbsp natural peanut butter	½ cup low-fat cottage cheese 1 tbsp natural peanut butter

Don't Neglect Proper Hydration

The importance of water cannot be stressed enough! Especially when you are involved in vigorous activities and lose water through sweat, you need to diligently replace your body's stores of liquid, preferably in the form of water. That can actually add up to **2 to 3 gallons (9 to 13 liters) of water per day when performing intense workouts!**

There are several reasons *why water is so important*:

- It provides the fluidity to blood to transport oxygen and nutrients
- Water helps regulate body temperature
- Hydration facilitates digestion and other body functions
- Water helps flush out and remove cellular wastes and toxins.

In the next chapter, HIIT as a tool for weight loss will be discussed.

A Word About Toxins

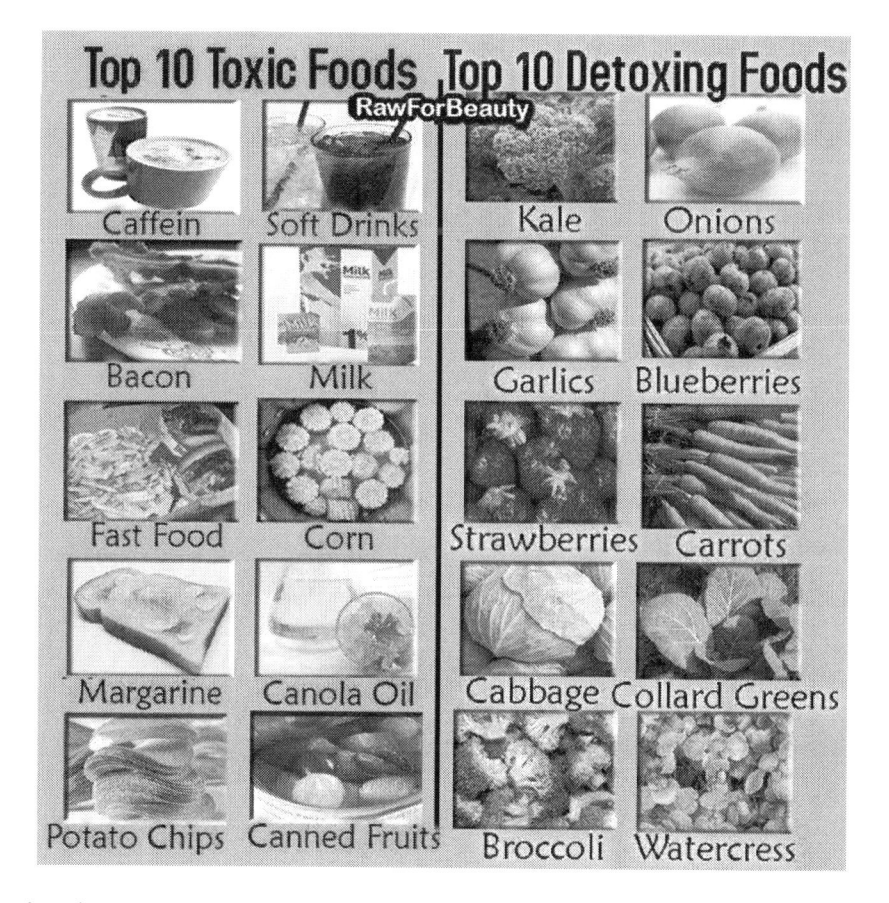

Top 10 Toxic Foods / Top 10 Detoxing Foods (RawForBeauty)

Toxic: Caffein, Soft Drinks, Bacon, Milk, Fast Food, Corn, Margarine, Canola Oil, Potato Chips, Canned Fruits

Detoxing: Kale, Onions, Garlics, Blueberries, Strawberries, Carrots, Cabbage, Collard Greens, Broccoli, Watercress

Another trendy topic is detoxification but just like with everything else, there are pros and cons. When it comes to increasing your activity level, though, it is an important concept. It does not mean that you have to spend days (or even just one) 'detoxing' but that you incorporate some of these ideas into your daily routine and eating habits.

The body detoxifies itself in several ways:

- Digestive tract

- Liver (to the blood stream)

- Kidneys (to the bladder)

- Respiratory system and lungs

- Lymphatic system

- Skin (through sweat)

Cellular function naturally creates wastes that must be removed but most toxins are stored in the fat of the body. It is easy to conclude, then, **that with less fat, the body will hold fewer toxins**. A detox diet does not do much to remove fat, however. The main result of such a treatment is the removal of water, excess carbohydrate stores and residual intestinal contents.

When the body begins to break down fats as a result of exercise, fat-soluble chemicals are released into the blood stream. In quantity, these toxins can make you feel tired, increase muscle soreness and even lead to nausea. This is why considering improving your body's ability to remove toxins is important when you start a diet and/or exercise program.

Detox adjustments to your diet may jump-start healthier body chemistry but maintaining proper nutrition and hydration promotes a permanent state of detox that leads to better health and a leaner, fitter body. Together with dietary improvements, regular HIIT workouts fine-tune the body's metabolism to function even more efficiently and improve overall cellular function.

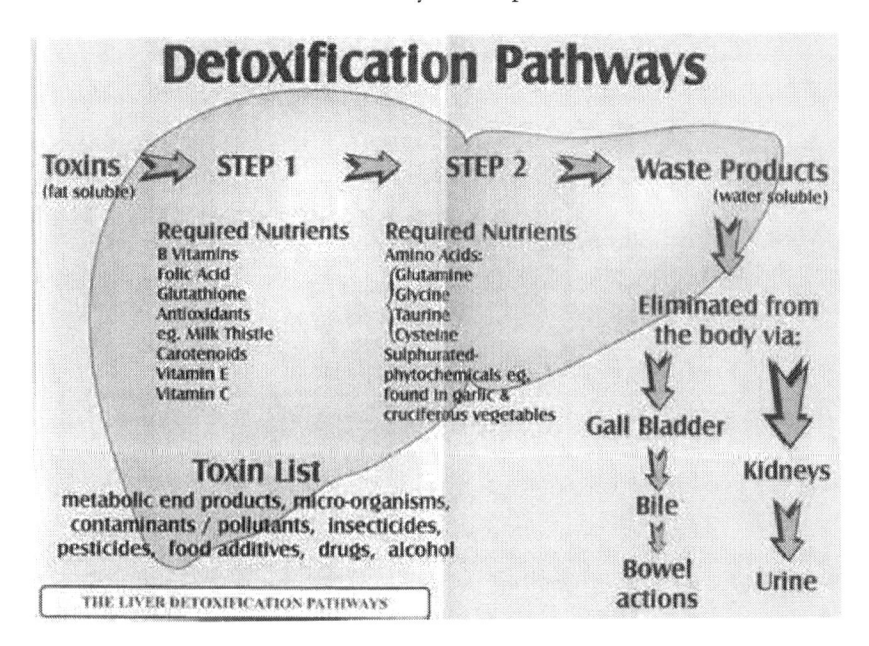

Detoxification Pathways

Toxins (fat soluble) ⇒ STEP 1 ⇒ STEP 2 ⇒ Waste Products (water soluble)

Step 1 Required Nutrients:
- B Vitamins
- Folic Acid
- Glutathione
- Antioxidants eg. Milk Thistle
- Carotenoids
- Vitamin E
- Vitamin C

Step 2 Required Nutrients:
Amino Acids:
- Glutamine
- Glycine
- Taurine
- Cysteine

Sulphurated phytochemicals eg. found in garlic & cruciferous vegetables

Toxin List: metabolic end products, micro-organisms, contaminants / pollutants, insecticides, pesticides, food additives, drugs, alcohol

Eliminated from the body via:
- Gall Bladder ⇒ Bile ⇒ Bowel actions
- Kidneys ⇒ Urine

THE LIVER DETOXIFICATION PATHWAYS

CHAPTER 4 – HIIT AND WEIGHT LOSS

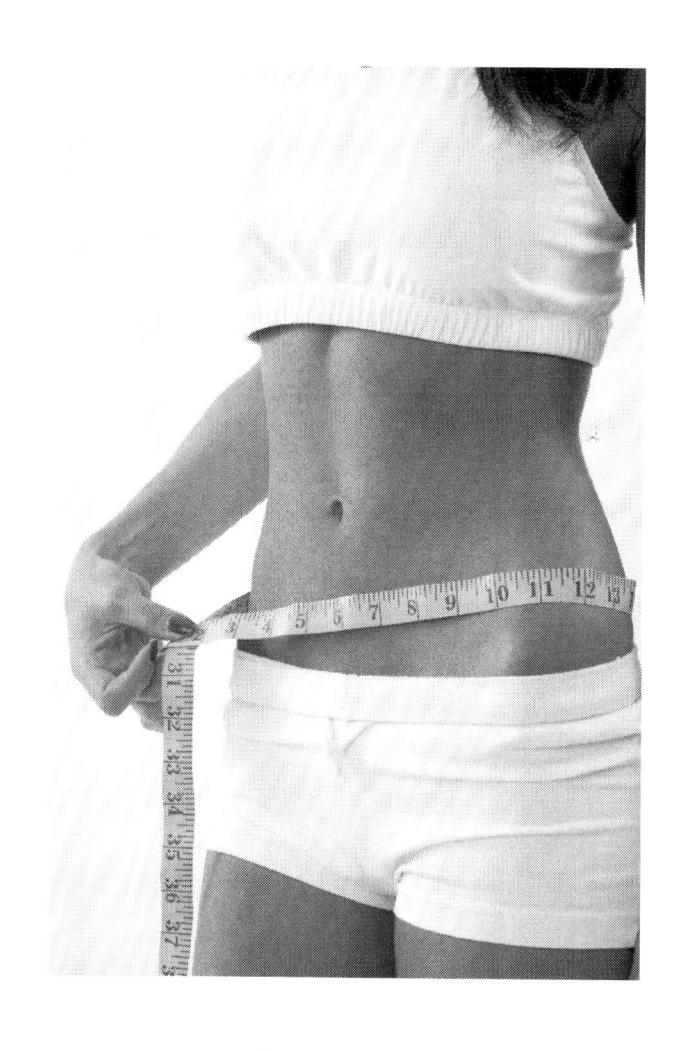

Everyone is looking for a magic pill, potion or program for easy weight loss and a killer body. The truth is there simply is no secret to success but **HIIT and a sensible diet are the closest you can come**.

Putting together the facts from Chapter 2 and Chapter 3, we come down to the reasons why HIIT is an excellent tool for weight loss. A HIIT workout is the ideal way to bring your body to the point of regular anaerobic metabolism so that glycolysis takes over to create the energy needed for continued cellular function.

The Body Becomes a Fat Burning Machine

Glucose is the primary source of fuel that powers the body. For the most part, it is a product of the digestion of carbohydrates, starch and sugars in the foods we eat, and is in abundant supply as long as there is oxygen present to help with the conversion to energy.

When the need for glucose surpasses what is available in circulation in the blood, reserves of glycogen that have been stored in the liver and muscles begin to break down to be converted to glucose.

After the body has used up glucose and glycogen, non-carbohydrate elements can be broken down to provide glucose. These elements include amino acids from proteins and glycerol from fat. It is possible for the body to use up almost all the fat stored in adipose tissues for the creation of energy in the absence of adequate glucose.

ATP, the energy from the metabolism of glucose, is continually produced during moderate exercise. As the heart rate and breathing rate increase, more oxygen is taken in and spread through the body to promote aerobic metabolism. When the demands on the body continue to the point where the lactate threshold is passed, the body automatically switches to anaerobic metabolism until the build-up of lactic acid prevents further activity.

The high intensity of HIIT workouts forces the body into the anaerobic mode, completely depleting the body's stores of glycogen in the cells of the muscles. The lower intensity or resting recovery periods provide the break the body needs for aerobic metabolism to break down fat and protein to create more carbohydrates that can then be converted into glucose.

It is through alternating high and low intensity workouts that the body is 'programmed' into burning fat during resting periods –12 and even up to 24 – 36 hours after the actual workout is complete – the After Burner Effect!

Fat Metabolism

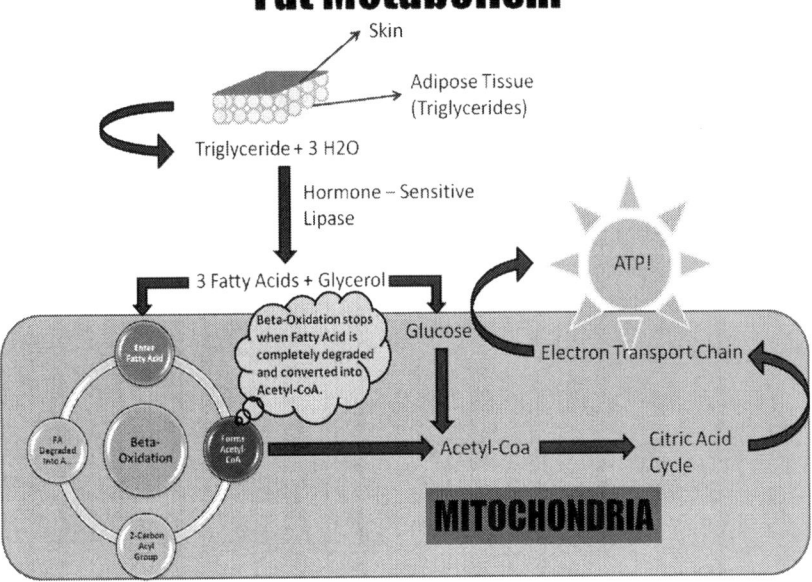

- Skin
- Adipose Tissue (Triglycerides)

Triglyceride + 3 H2O

Hormone-Sensitive Lipase

3 Fatty Acids + Glycerol

Glucose

ATP!

Electron Transport Chain

Beta-Oxidation cycle (MITOCHONDRIA):
- Enter Fatty Acid
- Beta-Oxidation
- Forms Acetyl-CoA
- 2-Carbon Acyl Group
- FA Degraded into A.

Beta-Oxidation stops when Fatty Acid is completely degraded and converted into Acetyl-CoA.

Acetyl-CoA → Citric Acid Cycle

HIIT Makes the Entire Body Work Hard

That may seem obvious but it means that along with the sweating and aching muscles, all the cellular processes within the body become involved and get a good workout. With the intense activity incorporated into a HIIT session, the **body reaches a number of critical thresholds that stimulate defensive reactions**:

- Reduced oxygen supply and increased blood carbon dioxide

- Increased body temperature

- Reduced available fuel stores – low blood sugar

- Reduced body fluids - dehydration

- Tissue damage – injury

In reacting to these danger signals, the body must adapt and that is where the **benefits of HIIT** are observed, especially **in respect to weight loss**.

- Reduction in body fat without losing muscle mass

- Strengthening of the cardiovascular system

- Increased 'work capacity' (tolerating more intensity for longer periods of time)

- Improved oxidation of carbohydrates and fat in skeletal muscle

- Challenging fast-twitch muscles (that build power, strength and physique)

- Improved mental attitude.

Lose Weight While You Rest

Now that sounds like magic! After a HIIT workout, your body continues to burn calories in order to return to its normal physiological and chemical resting state - *homeostasis*. This is the beauty of anaerobic metabolism! Glycogen does not need energy to be broken down for use by the cells but it needs energy to replenish the supply. In order for the blood sugar to be made available for the metabolic system of the muscles during periods of rest, energy is used and this is part of the 'after burner' effect.

Because of the tremendous demands created by HIIT activities, a suitable balance between supplying body needs (rest and carbohydrates) and expending energy (muscular and stress-related) is necessary for overall health and wellness. Stated another way, there has to be balance between activities involving the parasympathetic nervous system ('rest and digest') and the sympathetic nervous system ('fight or flight').

You **work hard for 20 to 30 minutes during a HIIT session** which is just up to the point of depletion of glycogen stores. **In the following hours**, your body converts fat to replenish that glucogen and **you lose weight while you are 'resting'**!

What About Calories?

Counting calories or trying to determine how many are being burned is a mental challenge that does not really prove much. Like so many things in life, it is all relative. What this means is that the total weight and fat vs. muscle composition of the body, intensity of activity, aerobic vs. anaerobic metabolism and nutrient sources available to the body are all factors that create different results for different individuals and even the same person on different days.

Given the body's need to protect itself – maintain homeostasis – some of what seems logical is, in fact, counter-productive. Cellular function and metabolic rate are set based on the availability of food. It is that plain and simple. If you reduce food intake, the body goes on the defensive and slows the metabolism so that it does not run out of fuel. When the metabolism slows down, it is harder to lose weight. That is why **crash dieting and severely limiting caloric intake result in increased weight gain when the 'diet' is over**!

If you increase your caloric needs by exercising, you actually need to have adequate calorie intake. The problem with most people, though, is that their calorie intake is already higher than their energy demands and the calories come from the wrong types of foods. Adopting a better overall diet will bring the available calories and nutrients into better alignment with the needs of the body.

For those of you who need to see some numbers, there are general rates for **caloric burn based on the intensity of the activity and the body weight of the person** involved. The heavier the person, the more calories will be burned performing the same activity for the same length of time.

Calories Burned per 30 Minutes of Activity at Your Weight

Activity Done for 30 Minutes at:	100 lbs	120 lbs	140 lbs	160 lbs	180 lbs	200 lbs	220 lbs	240 lbs	260 lbs	280 lbs
Aerobic Dancing	115	138	161	184	207	230	253	276	299	322
Aerobic Step Training	145	174	203	232	261	290	319	348	377	406
Backpacking (20 lb load)	200	240	280	320	360	400	440	480	520	560
Basketball	130	156	182	208	234	260	286	312	338	364
Bicycling	200	240	280	320	360	400	440	480	520	560
Dancing	100	120	140	160	180	200	220	240	260	280
Gardening	90	108	126	144	162	180	198	216	234	252
Golf, walking without cart	100	120	140	160	180	200	220	240	260	280
Housework	90	108	126	144	162	180	198	216	234	262
Jogging (5 mph)	185	222	259	296	333	370	407	444	481	518
Mowing	135	162	189	216	243	270	297	324	351	378
Skipping Rope	285	342	399	456	513	570	627	684	741	798
Stair Climber Machine	160	192	224	256	288	320	352	384	416	448
Swimming (25 yards per min)	120	144	168	192	216	240	264	288	312	336
Walking (15 minute mile)	100	120	140	160	180	200	220	240	260	280
Weight Training (90 seconds between sets)	125	150	175	200	225	250	275	300	325	350

These numbers are based on roughly 180 pounds of body weight.

- ✓ To burn 300 calories, you need to

    - Walk moderately for 1 hour with some inclines

    - Participate in a ballet class or barre workout for 1 hour

    - Weed a garden for 60 minutes

    - Bowl for 90 minutes (not counting waiting or marking down your score!)

    - Do HIIT for 20 minutes

- ✓ To burn 400 calories, you need to

    - Take a Zumba or similar dance workout class for 45 minutes

    - Engage in circuit training for 40 minutes

HIIT

- Run at roughly 7 mph for 35 minutes
- Play basketball for 35 minutes
- Do HIIT for 25 minutes

✓ To burn 500 calories, you need to
- Climb stairs for 40 minutes
- Perform kickboxing for 40 minutes
- Take a spin class for 40 minutes
- Swim laps vigorously for 35 minutes
- Do HIIT for 30 minutes

When and What to Eat?

Given the intensity of a HIIT workout, it is best to **eat a meal at least 1 to 1 ½ hours before exercising**. Not only do you want to give the food a chance to pass through the stomach to avoid nausea, it needs to be digesting so that the nutrients are available as soon as the workout is over.

Also, **do not eat immediately after your session** because you don't want simple carbohydrates available for quick conversion to energy while the 'after burn' effect is working at its maximum. In half an hour or a little longer after working out, a protein-based snack or shake is the best boost for your body.

Numerous small meals are better than 3 regular meals when it comes to providing an even fuel supply for intense muscle workouts. That does not mean a wide range of foods at each time, but more of a **healthy snack interspersed in between regular meals**. It comes down to a matter of personal choice, circumstances and convenience. The crucial point, though, is the quality and variety of the food that is consumed (and that was covered in Chapter 3).

3 Meals a Day (BAD)

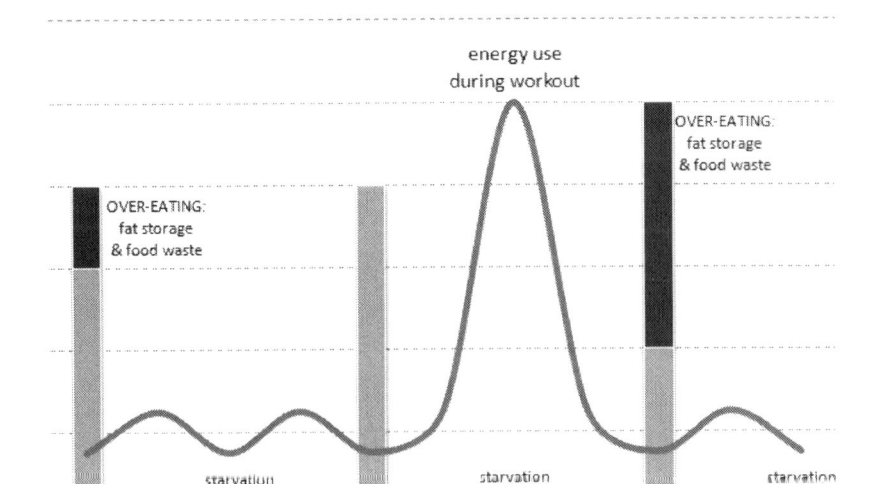

6 Meals a Day (GOOD)

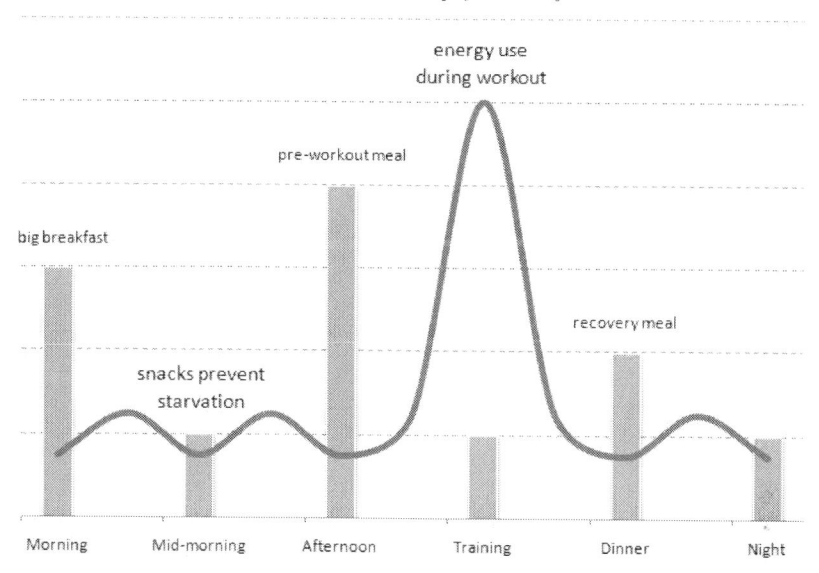

Chart showing energy distribution across six meals: Morning (big breakfast), Mid-morning (snacks prevent starvation), Afternoon (pre-workout meal), Training (energy use during workout), Dinner (recovery meal), Night.

As a general rule, it is best to **consume more carbohydrates on HIIT activity days than on non-intense training days**. Adequate hydration is always important and the addition of electrolytes can help recovery. After a HIIT workout, drinking a whey powder shake can replace some protein that could be lost to glycolysis.

Targeting Those 'Problem Areas'

Even with overall weight loss, there are still some parts of the body that tend to be more resistant to change. That can be addressed with exercises that focus on those areas during HIIT workouts and the result will include better sculpting and firmness. It is important to **maintain proper form and technique for both compound and isolation movements**, especially during higher intensity, to avoid injury.

The most common body-shape complaint is abdominal visceral fat – **'belly fat'**. The intensity of HIIT and the metabolic reaction to the demands of this activity combine to attack belly fat fast. In the next chapter, we will be looking at cardio routines to use as a basis for HIIT workouts and include a set of tips for targeting belly fat.

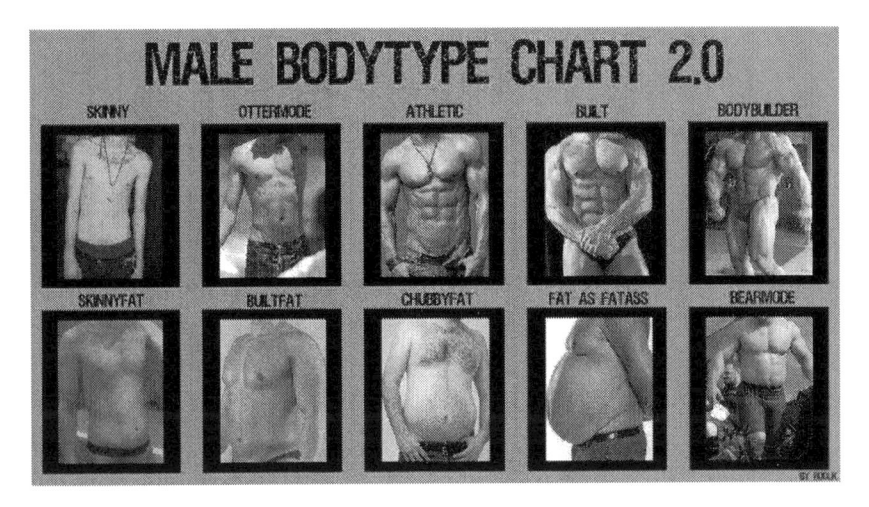

CHAPTER 5 – HIIT AND CARDIO

There is absolutely no denying the fact that cardio workouts **benefit the body in terms of overall fitness and cardiovascular health**. By changing a traditional Low Intensity Steady State (LISS) cardio session into a HIIT workout, you maximize the benefits and minimize the time commitment. In other words, you can spend 45 minutes to an hour 5 days a week or work harder for 20 to 30 minutes, 3 days a week for even better results.

HIIT cardio is also a better choice for most people compared to steady state cardio since it **burns fat without turning to protein synthesis for energy**. Just compare pictures of marathon runners and sprinters to see which type of body you prefer!

Which body is best for health and performance?

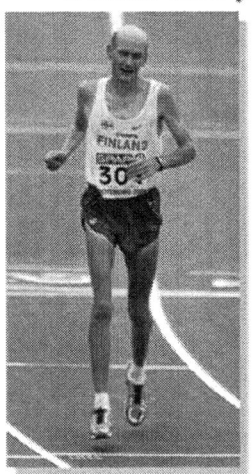

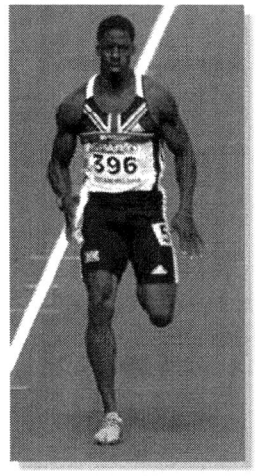

Make Any Cardio Activity a HIIT Cardio Workout

Variety is the spice of life and so it goes with exercise routines as well. Repeating the same activity over and over leads to boredom and limits the muscle groups that supply the work. By mixing up your cardio activities, you maintain a positive attitude towards your workout and create a better, more evenly toned body.

There is no set routine for any HIIT workout – it can be whatever you choose. Try a few options, see what works best for you and fill out a plan of action from there. It can simply be cardio or include aspect of cross-training, endurance or weight lifting, all of which are discussed in subsequent chapters.

For any HIIT cardio workout, you need to **begin with a simple 5 minute warm up** to get your body ready for the hard stuff.

Remember, **the key to HIIT workouts is to alternate high intensity work and moderate intensity recovery** over the entire 10 to 20 minute workout. Choosing the 'right' intervals is a matter of personal choice based on fitness level – that is why HIIT is great for individuals of all ages and abilities! You do what is comfortable for you just as long as you are hitting close to 90% effort during the intense sections of the intervals and dropping down to no more than 60% effort during the recovery phases.

Examples of the *most common work/recovery intervals* (easier to harder) are:

Sample Intervals for HIIT Workouts

(work seconds / recovery seconds)

- **Easier**
  10/30
  15/45
  30/90
  60/180
  90/270

120/360

- **Harder**
  10/20
  15/30
  30/60
  60/120
  90/180
  120/240

- **Hardest**
  10/10
  15/15
  30/30
  60/60
  90/90
  120/120

- **Killer**
  10/5
  15/8
  30/15
  60/30
  90/45
  120/60

For the best workout, the intervals used can be varied for more of a challenge to the metabolic pathways. **After some short intervals, do some longer intervals and continue to switch it up** while maintaining a steady work to recovery ratio. For example, progress through the increased times of the easier column or shorten recovery intervals after the same work intervals.

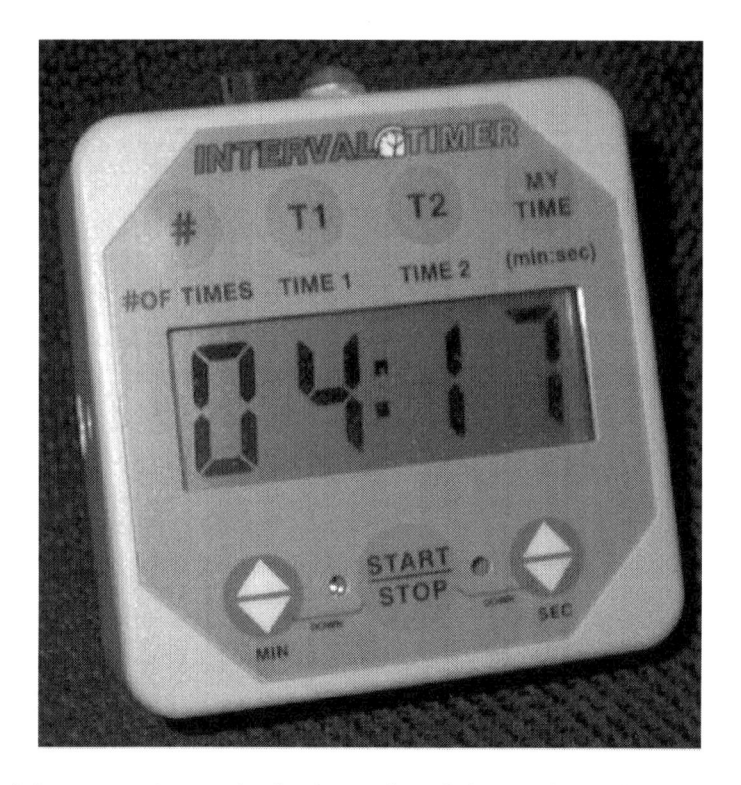

It can't be repeated enough: **the intensity of the work portion of the session is the key**. You should not exceed 90 to 95% of maximum heart rate and certainly drop it down a notch or two if you become dizzy or lightheaded. Working over 95% of HR max may not leave you with enough energy to complete a full 20 to 30 minute HIIT session.

On the other hand, you can tell if you have not worked hard enough if you are not still sweating for at least 10 minutes after the session, if you are regularly performing 1 and 2 minute high intensity bursts or it seems that you could keep working out after a 20 minute session (unless you are super-fit and normally perform 30 minute sessions).

Sample Cardio Workouts

Bicycling: Adjust the seat so that your legs are not quite completely extended. Hold the handle bar gently but securely and crouch slightly forward. Don't strain against the handlebar - you are simply using it for balance.

Cardio Kickboxing: Starting with some stretches and a brief cardio warm up, cardio kickboxing takes a number of forms that incorporate resistance training and circuit training using heavy bags, training pads or martial arts movements. A full body workout can be achieved at a gym or at home.

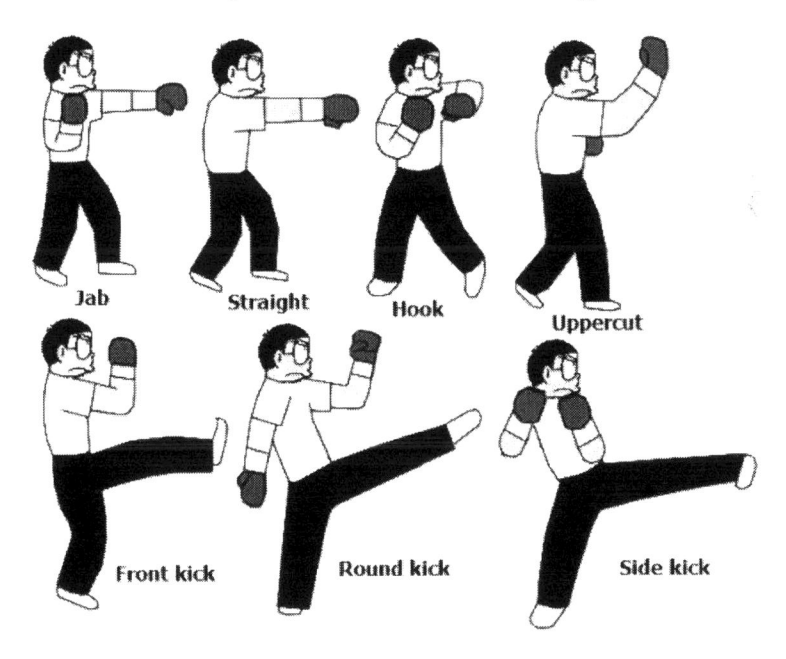

Elliptical Machine: This is a great full-body workout since both the legs and arms are involved. Complete 8 to 10 sets of 60/60 intervals with a 5 minute warm up and 5 minute cool down or stretches for a great basic cardio workout. Simply let your body work in sync with the machine for a manual or programmed exercise session. Keep your shoulders loose and your core firm. Be sure to warm up and cool down to prevent injuries. For more intensity, add elevation or wear extra weight.

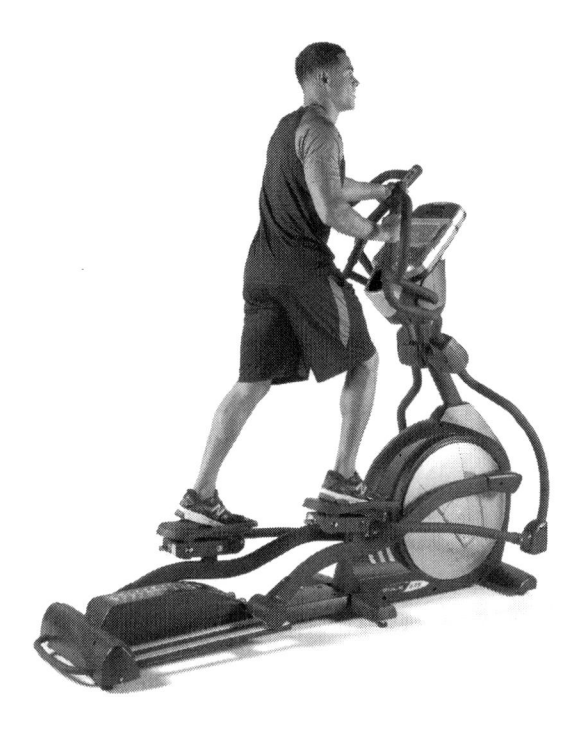

Jumping Rope: If you're sure you won't tie yourself up in the rope, jumping rope (with the single foot method as if you are running in place) is an easy way to reach maximum intensity. After 60 seconds of high intensity, slow down for the next 60 seconds and work through 10 or 12 sets for a total of 20 to 25 minutes. Keeping your elbows in and forearms parallel to the floor, turn the rope with your wrists and forearms. Since this is pretty tough on knees and ankles, jump rope on a rubber gym floor or some other padded surface. To determine the right length of rope, stand on the rope and hold the handles up roughly to your armpits.

Roller Blading: Smoother and easier on the joints than running, inline skating provides a complete aerobic and anaerobic workout that improves overall endurance, cardiovascular function, flexibility and strength. Greater use of inner thigh and buttock muscles than required for most other activities helps those 2 problem areas.

Running: Feet should follow a straight line and arms should swing gently front to back, mostly from the elbow. Brace your core and don't lean forward as you run to avoid stress on the lower back.

Spinning: Spinning or working out on a stationary bike allows you to set the speed and resistance. When you begin to go too fast on a bike, you risk losing control so increasing resistance as you become accustomed to the workout helps you maintain the intensity.

Sprinting: If you have access to a track or a safe stretch of road, sprinting is a terrific way to build up cardio out in the fresh air. Finding a hill to run up then walk down is the perfect way to increase intensity. With the intensity of the HIIT workout, though, sprinting is hard on the knees and other leg joints.

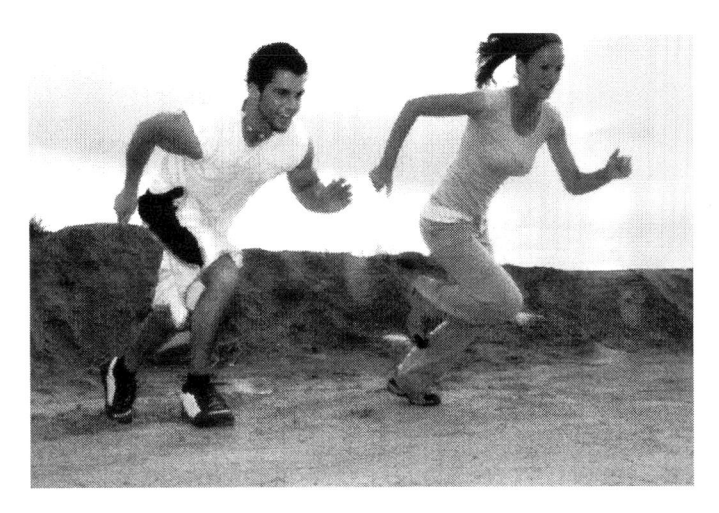

Stair Running: Indoors or outdoors, running up stairs for 60 seconds is extremely demanding. Walk back down for 60 seconds then run back up. Make sure there are several flights since you won't cover the same distance up and down!

Swimming: Follow the same procedure as for the other cardio workouts by warming up then alternating intense swimming for 60 seconds with treading water for 60 seconds. This is an excellent exercise to target the whole body – arms, legs and core - with reaching and stretching for each stroke.

Treadmill: When a track or open road is not available, a treadmill can provide the same sprinting options. After 5 minutes warming up, set the speed to an all-out run for 60 seconds then bring it down to a jog for the next 60 seconds. Be careful of the possibility of falling off, though! 8 to 10 sets should have the heart pumping and the sweat pouring off, but don't forget to cool down.

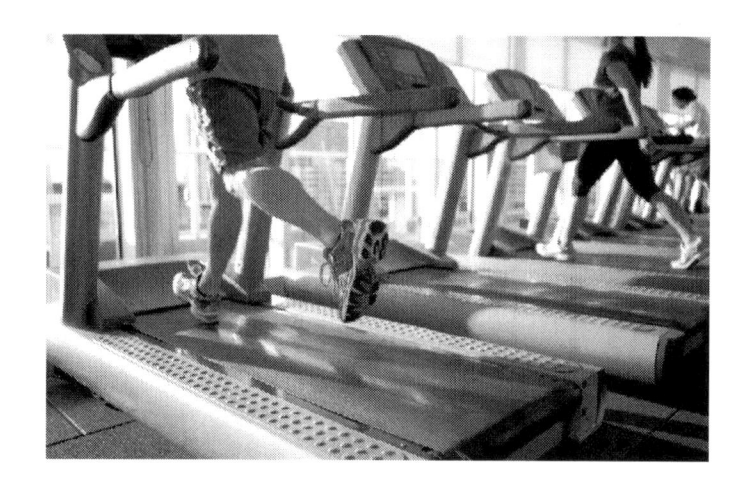

CHAPTER 6 – HIIT AND CROSS-TRAINING

To overcome the effects of specificity – working only a particular set of muscles related to a specific activity – **aerobic, strength training and flexibility exercises were added to workout routines** and cross training was developed.

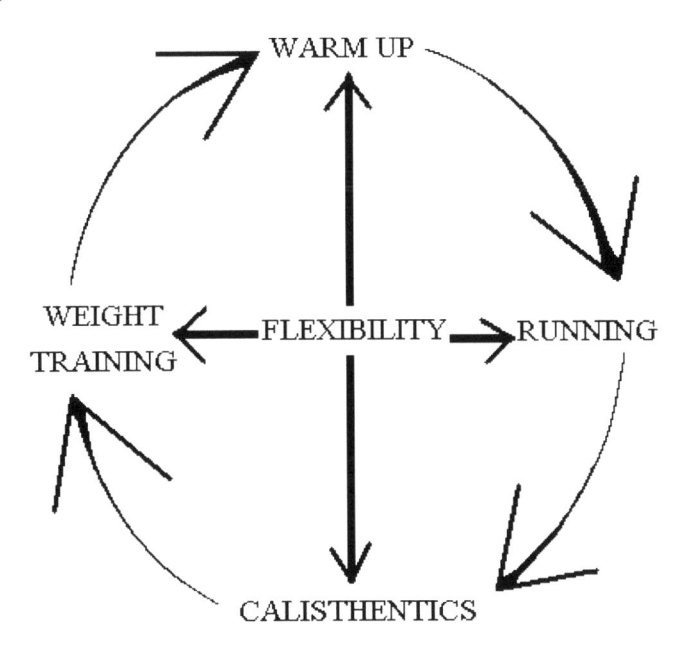

Cross training has become quite popular throughout the various sport and fitness disciplines **for a variety of reasons**:

- Toning and conditioning all muscles, tendons and joints for balanced physical ability and improved strength, speed and agility

- Reducing the risk of injury by incorporating all muscle groups with a wider range of motion instead of over-working certain ones

- Improving overall fat reduction by burning more calories

- Increasing cardio-vascular capability

- Maintaining muscle mass

- Removing boredom from over-used workout routines.

Any cross training activity can be incorporated into HIIT sessions which serve to intensify the benefits you get from your workout.

Cross Training Workouts

Cross training provides many different options for exercises that are fun and can be done in a wide range of circumstances. While most people think of running, cycling and swimming, there are plenty of other choices, both indoor and outdoor, to add tremendous variety to your overall arsenal of workout options. Instead of straight cardio, many people appreciate the ability to turn regular activities into HIIT workouts.

Core Strength Training: Similar to yoga in that you can increase muscle strength and flexibility, core strength training (whether through bodyweight exercises or machines) focuses on the muscles that stabilize the spine and allow for the efficient transfer of power to the legs and arms.

- **Bicycle Crunch**

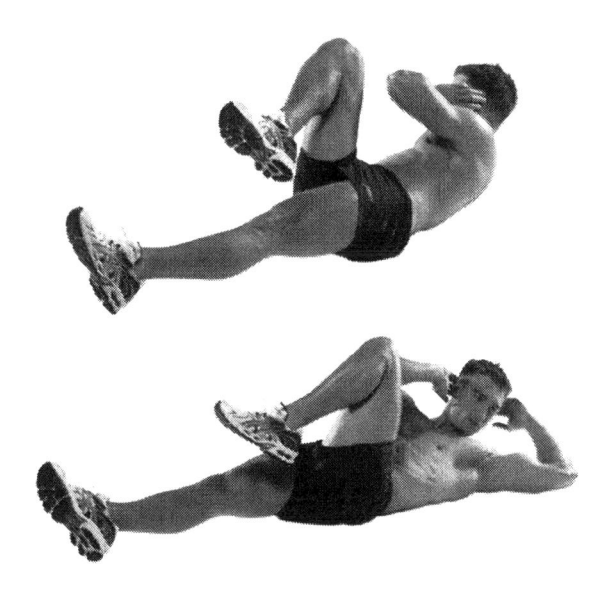

- **Bridge**

- **Single Leg Bridge**

- **Lunge**

- **Jump Lunge**

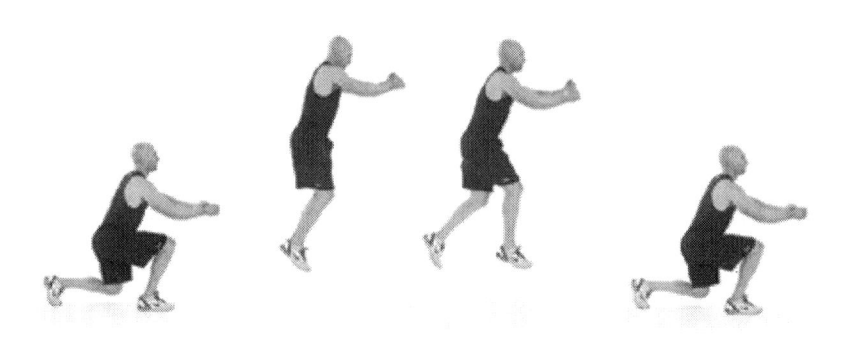

- **Plank and Side Plank**

- **Push Up Lat Row**

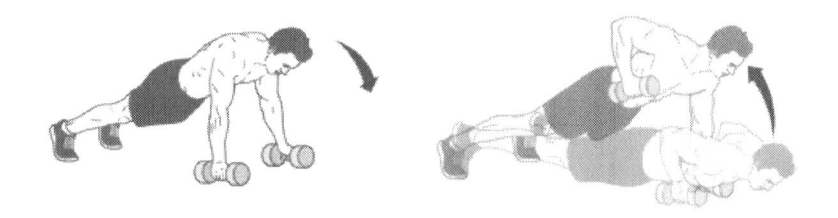

- **Skip with Twist**

- **V-Sit Abdominal Exercise**

HIIT

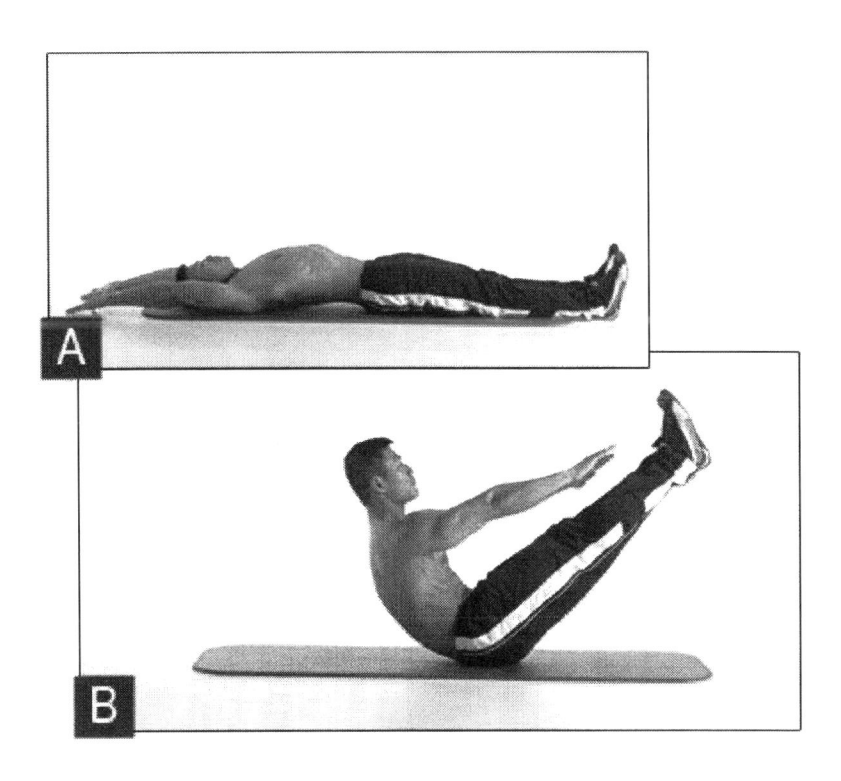

- Squat to knee lift twist

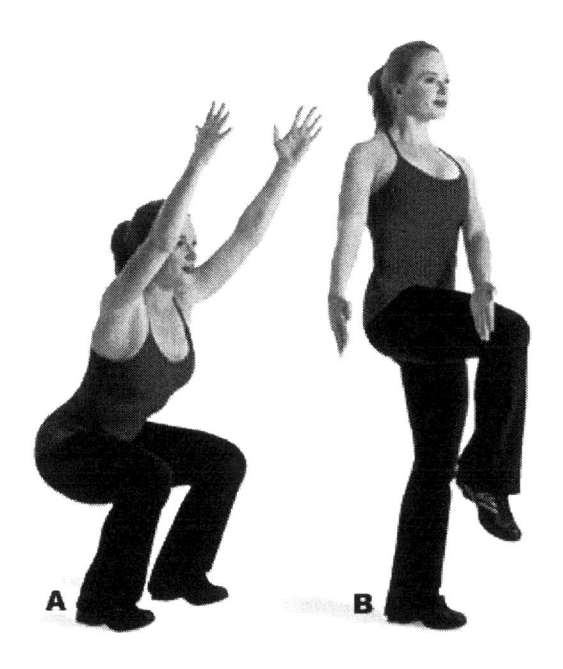

- Squat jump

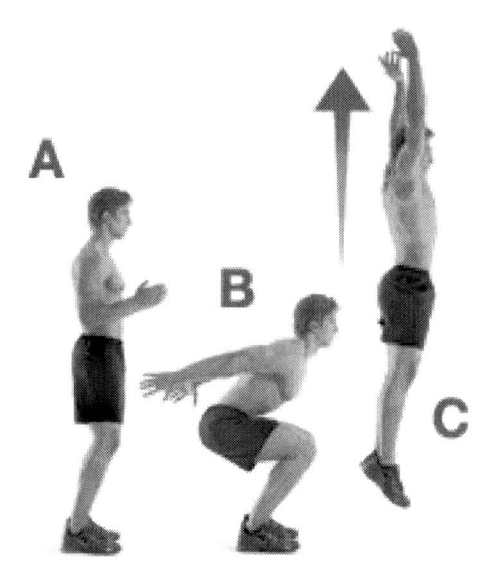

- Side leap and balance

- Crossing climber

- Standing straight leg bicycle

Muscles of the Core

A. Serratus anterior
B. Transverse abdominal
C. Internal oblique
D. External oblique
E. Aponeurosis of the ext. oblique
F. Linea alba
G. Tendinous insertion
H. Rectus abdominus

When you do your core exercises, these are the muscles that are strengthened. Major muscles of the core are shown above. They include muscles of the pelvic floor, lower back and diaphragm (not shown).

The Heart of the Core

The transverse abdominal – deep muscle of the core – wraps around the trunk like a corset. It attaches the lower ribs, diaphragm and lumbar spine to the hips. In effect, it ties the rib cage and upper body to the pelvis and lower body. It keeps you "connected."

The core stabilizes the body, protects the spinal column and provides a firm support for the various physical activities we perform.

Cross Country Skiing: Another full-body workout, cross country skiing uses all the muscles of the body with tremendous intensity that demands the highest degree of breathing efficiency. It doesn't take much to hit the full-on effort for HIIT and even the recovery periods are not easy!

Deep-Water Running: As a variation of pounding the pavement, deep water running offers all the benefits without the stress to joints and bones. This type of routine can actually replace running training in the event of injury since there is completely non-weight bearing. While wearing a flotation belt, you can imitate the motion of cross country skiing or simply alternately raising your knees as quickly as possible. For added intensity, remove the flotation belt so you have to work harder to stay above water.

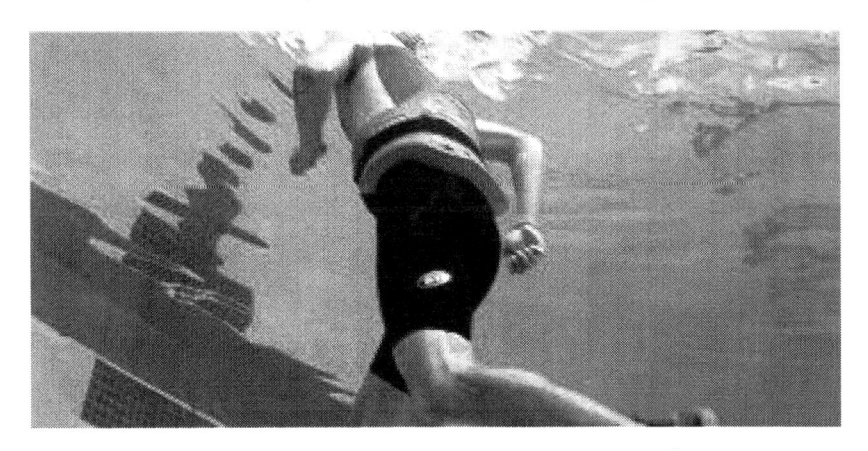

Kayaking: Core and upper body strength are the keys to successful kayaking. Adjusting power and speed are easy to do so a kayak trip can be a great HIIT cross training activity as well as a steady state cardio activity for non-intense workout days.

Kickboxing: Like aerobic dance, kickboxing provides a full body workout with attention to specific movements and muscle groups. With or without a heavy bag, the action of punching and kicking requires balance and a well-toned core and developing speed increases the intensity.

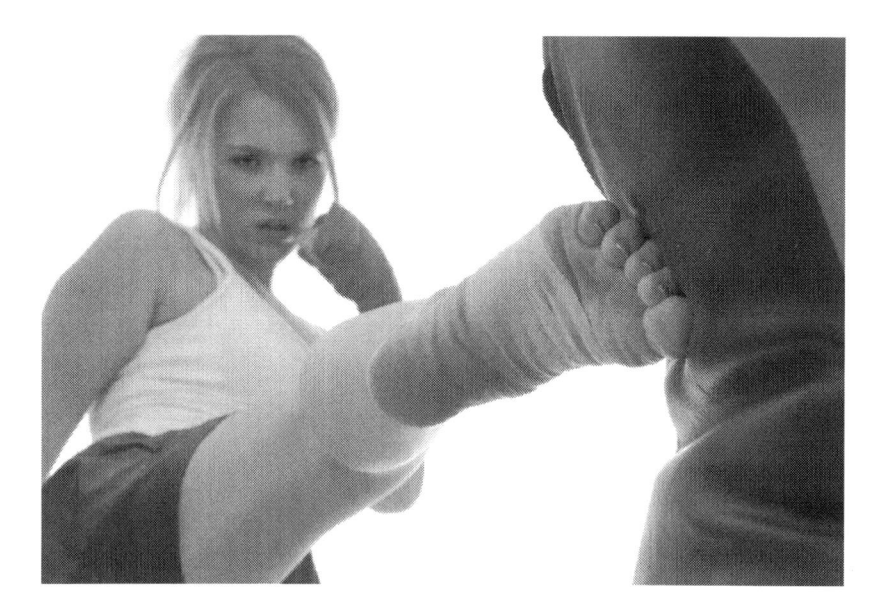

Pilates: Pilates is well-known for improved core strength and overall flexibility. A generalization describing Pilates as a **combination of yoga and core strength training** takes into account the functional nature of the exercise motions – lifting, leaning, pulling and pushing – along with concentrating on breathing and controlled movements. With or without equipment, Pilates workouts promote long, lean muscles with better posture and balance as well as increased lung and breathing capacity.

Rowing: Rowing machines or boats on the water provide a full-body workout demanding equal effort from both the upper and lower body. Maintain good form with a slightly rounded back and bringing your knees almost straight on the back stroke with your shoulder blades squeezed together as you pull the handle to your sternum.

Yoga: While most people think of yoga as a way to meditate and relax, there are numerous forms that require high intensity that improves breathing technique and facilitates the mind-body connection for better performance. Many of the yoga poses can be used to build strength and the full-body benefits include reduction in the discomfort of delayed onset muscle soreness (DOMS) after strenuous workouts.

Scheduling Cross Training Sessions

Timing is everything, especially when you are incorporating HIIT workouts into your weekly exercise plan. Because of the intense demands of HIIT activities, they should only be **performed 3 times in a week**. For maximum benefit, the types of exercises you incorporate into these workouts need to be dissimilar and planned out as well to avoid over-working some muscles and allowing all systems to have adequate rest and recovery to prevent over-training or CNS fatigue.

Research shows that **long workouts (cardio) are more efficient in the morning after a light meal**. The body has just had plenty of rest and is working on a fasting type of metabolism so fat burning is easier to achieve.

On the other hand, **intense workouts** such as sprints or race speed swimming **have better results in the afternoon** when the body has been fully warmed up from daytime activities and carbohydrate stores have been replenished through meals.

Choosing HIIT Workout Activities

Major muscle groups, particularly in the legs, contain the greatest number of mitochondria and are therefore the best to **focus on for the work intervals of your routine**. Many combinations are possible in a circuit training format so that you can address quite a few different skills in each workout such as cardio and strength training.

Another element to consider when choosing HIIT activities is the need for equipment. Working with a medicine ball, resistance bands or weights may require going to a gym while body weight activities and cardio can be done anywhere. **Burpees** are a great full-body, intense workout that can be combined with strength training exercises that alternate between the muscles of the legs, back, shoulders and arms.

Sample HIIT Workout Progression

Week	Warm-up	Work Interval (Max Intensity)	Recovery Interval (60-70% MHR)	Repeat	Cool Down	Total Workout Time
1	5 min.	30 sec.	2 min.	2 times	5 min.	15 min.
2	5 min.	30 sec.	2 min.	3 times	5 min.	17.5 min.
3	5 min.	30 sec.	2 min.	4 times	5 min.	20 min.
4	5 min.	1 min.	4 min.	2 times	5 min.	20 min.
5	5 min.	1 min.	4 min.	3 times	5 min.	25 min.
6	5 min.	1 min.	4 min.	4 times	5 min.	30 min.
7	5 min.	1.5 min.	4 min.	2 times	5 min.	21 min.
8	5 min.	1.5 min.	4 min.	3 times	5 min.	26.5 min.
9	5 min.	1.5 min.	4 min.	4 times	5 min.	32 min.
10	5 min.	2 min.	5 min.	2 times	5 min.	24 min.
11	5 min.	2 min.	5 min.	3 times	5 min.	31 min.

Variations in **heart rate** should be roughly between 175 bpm during work intervals and 100 – 110 bpm during recovery intervals. *The Borg Rating of Perceived Exertion Scale* is another way to determine intensity with numbers between 6 (no exertion) and 20 (maximum exertion). HIIT work intervals should be performed at roughly 17 to 19 and recovery intervals at about 11 – 13 for a relatively healthy individual. (It could be noted that there is a general correlation between the intensity level of the Borg Scale and heart rate when the RPE is multiplied by 10. For example, a Borg rating of 12 would mean a HR of 120 BPM.)

HIIT's unique features require everyone to *start slowly until the program is understood*. Adjusting the times is easy, though, for people of all fitness levels and abilities:

To make it more gradual

- Start with 15 second / 1 minute intervals with 2 reps, increasing to 3 and 4 reps

- Spend 2 weeks at each level instead of 1

- Add 30 seconds to the recovery time for each additional rep (i.e. 2 reps – 2 min., 3 reps – 2 min. 30 seconds, 3 reps- 3 min.)

- Add another 2 minutes to the cool down at a slightly lower intensity

To increase the intensity

- Start with 3 reps instead of 2 at each level

- Decrease recovery interval time to as little as half of the work interval time

- Increase intensity – run up-hill, increase resistance on the bike or treadmill, add weight.

When changing HIIT workout intervals, it is important to only change one at a time. What this means is that you can lengthen the work interval on a given level but keep the recovery interval the same. Similarly, decreases the recovery interval but maintain the same work interval.

(Remember – *Tabata style HIIT intervals* are set at 20 seconds work and 10 seconds of rest for the maximum workout you can achieve!)

CHAPTER 7 – HIIT AND ENDURANCE

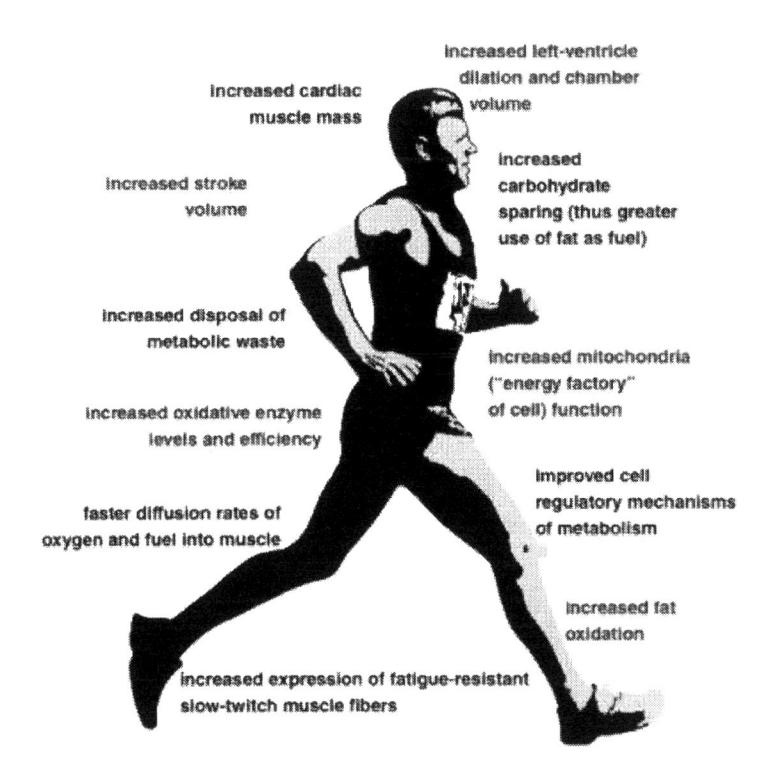

increased left-ventricle dilation and chamber volume

increased cardiac muscle mass

increased stroke volume

increased carbohydrate sparing (thus greater use of fat as fuel)

increased disposal of metabolic waste

increased mitochondria ("energy factory" of cell) function

increased oxidative enzyme levels and efficiency

improved cell regulatory mechanisms of metabolism

faster diffusion rates of oxygen and fuel into muscle

increased fat oxidation

increased expression of fatigue-resistant slow-twitch muscle fibers

According to the *Medical Dictionary for the Health Professions and Nursing* © *Farlex 2012*, **'Endurance' is the ability of both cardiac or skeletal muscles and the entire musculoskeletal system to sustain or generate a force over a period of time**. That is why athletes train – to improve upon the ability of their muscles and bodily systems.

What Is Improved Endurance?

Long term endurance (like marathon running) depends on aerobic metabolism and is a product of general cardiovascular fitness and the supply of glycogen available to the muscles for fuel.

Short term endurance can refer to local muscular endurance (such as weight lifting) where cardiovascular is not so important or to anaerobic endurance in which the whole body is involved in short bursts of activity at tremendous intensity (such as sprints).

Although both types of endurance are quite different in practice, they both depend on the same thing – a well-trained, fit body that has been 'fine-tuned' to optimize metabolic processes.

Traditionally speaking, increasing the volume of continuous aerobic exercise is the best way to improve overall cardiovascular fitness. This is due to the fact that heart performance is affected by aerobic exercise in a positive way so that the overall blood flow and oxygen supply can be increased and efficiently moved to satisfy the demands of the muscles.

Not only does aerobic exercise improve heart rate, stroke volume and heart contractility, the skeletal muscles do their part by boosting the preload of the heart. In other words, the venous blood (that is returning to the heart) is propelled by stronger skeletal muscle contractions and fills the ventricle more so the heart works more efficiently under stress, more blood is pumped per beat and each contraction of the heart muscle is more forceful.

Progressive endurance training is designed to cause adaptations to the actual heart muscle. The left ventricle expands to hold more blood and the muscle thickens to produce greater pumping strength. This type of adaptation usually occurs after regular aerobic training such as continuous running or cycling for at least 30 to 60 minutes.

How HIIT Benefits Overall Endurance

In a nutshell, **adding HIIT workouts to a traditional continuous endurance training routine provides the same benefits in less time**. For event training, you need to perform 'dress rehearsal' runs at a competitive level but for off-season or general training, HIIT offers equal physical gains with much greater diversity for better full-body fitness.

Many different studies have shown similar if not greater *improvements in VO2 max*, *cardio enhancement* such as heart stroke volume and ventricle size, and the *increase in the size and number of mitochondria* with HIIT workouts in comparison to standard endurance training.

How to Calculate your VO2 Max

Option 1: Resting Heart Rate Test
VO2 Max = 15.3 x (MHR/RHR)

MHR = Maximum Heart Rate = 208 − (0.7 x age)
RHR = Resting Heart Rate (take immediately upon waking up) = # of heartbeats in 1 minute

Option 2: Rockport Fitness Walking Test
Directions: walk 1 mile as fast as possible then take your HR for 10 seconds immediately after
VO2 Max = 132.853 − (0.0769 x W) − (0.3877 x A) + (6.315 x G) − (3.2649 x T) − (0.1565 X H)

W = Weight in pounds
A = Age
G = Gender. 0 for Females and 1 for Males.
T = Time to walk 1 mile
H = number of heartbeats in 10 seconds at the end of the walk

It is interesting to note that the metabolic adaptations regarding mitochondria and energy production utilize different message signaling pathways in HIIT training so that there is actually an *increase in fatty acid oxidation and EPOC* for a longer, *more efficient calorie burn after exercise.*

What this means to any athlete or fitness enthusiast is that the training program can be improved by adding HIIT workouts to the traditional endurance exercise routine.

By substituting HIIT several times a week, you save time while creating more toned muscle and greater metabolic efficiency.

You also get to vary your routine so that it is more enjoyable and interesting.

HIIT Programs for Different Types of Endurance

Depending on your fitness goals, you can choose between 2 types of HIIT sessions. The difference is simply a matter of timing since HIIT can be comprised of many different types of exercises.

For a 'power athlete', the goal is to improve anaerobic conditioning for better bursts of strength. The HIIT interval timing in this case should involve short 'work' intervals of no more than 30 seconds with an intensity of 90 – 100% of max.

The 'endurance athlete' needs to maintain excellent aerobic function so the 'work' interval should last longer than 30 seconds and up to several minutes with an intensity that requires from 80 – 100% of VO2 max.

In either case, the recovery intervals can reflect overall fitness and be varied to target specific energy systems. **Endurance intervals** of 1/1 or 1/2 and **power intervals** of 2/1 are typical.

How Much is Too Much?

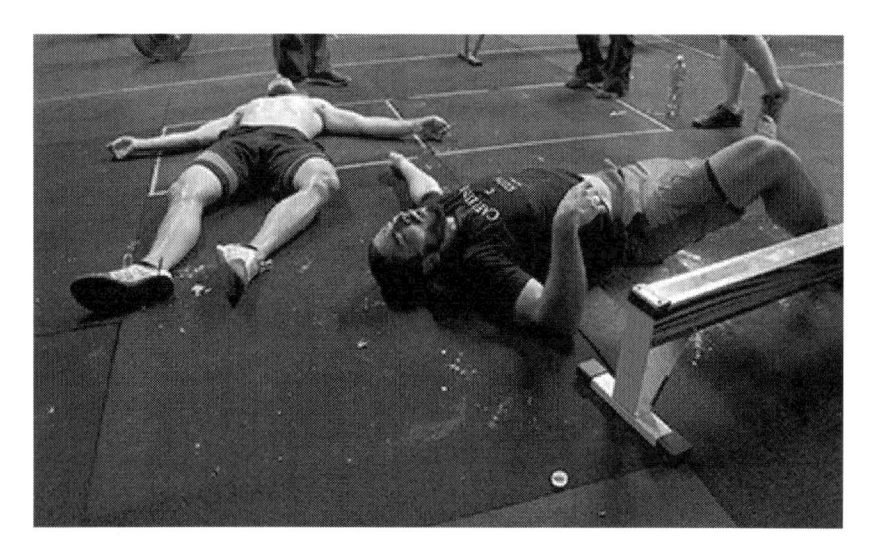

Just as important as knowing how to exercise for maximum benefit is knowing when to stop to prevent injury or CNS fatigue. A common question from intense athletes involves **how often HIIT can be performed in the course of a week** and **if it can be done with other workout sessions**.

Let's just look at some basic facts and you can begin to see the answer clearly for yourself.

1. HIIT workouts should be so intense that you are completely exhausted.

2. HIIT recovery intervals and cool down are absolutely necessary and cannot be avoided. Even if you are too tired to cool down, you don't want to risk blood pooling in your extremities!

3. Heart rate should drop to 70% of max during recovery.

4. Fatigue or soreness means that your body is demanding rest – it has been depleted and needs to recover.

5. For beginners, the work to rest interval should be roughly 1/4 – it takes that long for the body to adjust itself to the demands.

6. Progressive overload – increasing the volume, intensity and fre-

quency of training – is progressive based on the body's reaction to the demands, not according to the calendar or a schedule.

Overtraining Syndrome was discussed in Chapter 2 - The Science Behind HIIT and offers more details about the effects of too much stress on the body. Let's just repeat here that overtraining means not being able to handle the workout load *you usually can* and feeling tired, dissatisfied and in discomfort. It's about regression – losing the gains you have made.

HIIT workouts are all about intensity and timing and the **general recommendation is to perform them only 3 times per week**. The other days can be used for cardio training that strictly target aerobic fitness or strength training that is primarily anaerobic.

There are ways, however, **to incorporate HIIT activities on a more frequently basis** without hitting the proverbial wall. The key is to *choose activities that are as different as possible* – using different muscle groups – *and keeping the overall reps to a minimum for a shorter workout time*. For example, if you cycle one day, row the next, swim another and do calisthenics the next.

Rest Days Are Critical To Overall Performance!

- Repair tissue

- Replenish energy stores

- Decrease risk of injury

- Prevent burnout

CHAPTER 8 – HIIT AND WEIGHT LIFTING

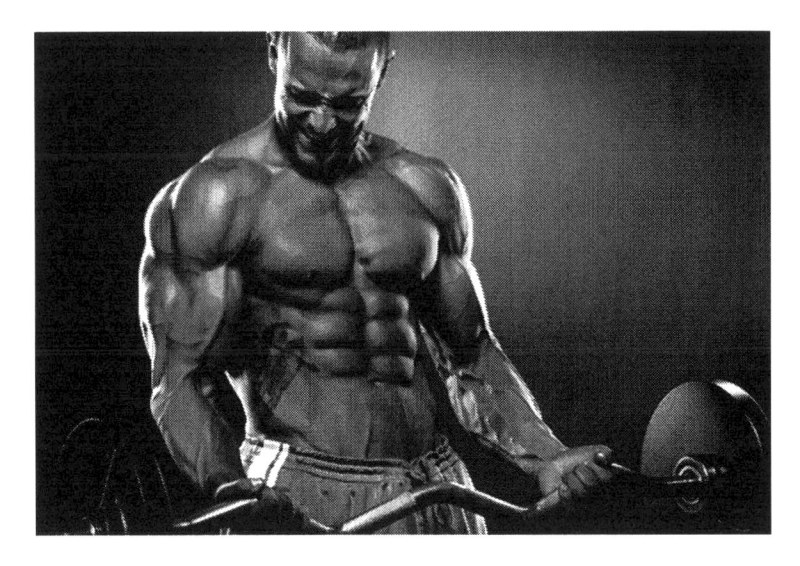

The physical demands of **weight lifting and** the intensity of **HIIT** workouts are similar and **are best done on different days**. The drain on energy during either activity does not leave adequate reserves for the optimum performance of the other on the same day, even after a period of rest – but it is all relative to overall fitness, the choice of activities and timing. HIIT workouts can be done once a week and still provide benefits to body builders preparing for competition but during the 'off' season, HIIT can be done 3 times per week on alternate days with weight training in between.

Incorporating HIIT into a Weight Lifting Regimen

While most weight lifters and trainers would normally avoid cardio training since it tends to break down muscle mass. After 45 minutes, catabolic (anaerobic) metabolism kicks in and utilizes the protein from muscles for fuel. It has been found that **HIIT cardio workouts enhance the body's ability to build muscle mass** since it turns to fat for anaerobic fuel. (Again, consider the appearance of marathon runners and sprinters!).

In reality, weight lifting is a type of HIIT workout since it involves anaerobic respiration so why would other HIIT disciplines hurt! Based on what you have read so far in this book, you should be thinking that very same thing. A HIIT workout puts maximum stress on the body/muscles/metabolism in a short period of time and by varying the form of the workout, you can target the whole body for better overall fitness and function while preventing injury or overload. Weight lifting is rather limited in terms of range of motion and the incorporation of multiple muscle groups so alternating strength workouts with HIIT training is the best of both worlds.

Essentially, by incorporating HIIT activities into your weight lifting routine, you will receive **the benefits from both interval training and weight training**:

- Building muscles and lean tissue (remember the mitochondria!)

- Increasing your ability to burn fat

- Increasing glycogen stored in the muscles for more readily available fuel

- Increasing hypertrophy by raising the concentration of myofibrillar nuclei.

Each workout is made up of 3 distinct elements:

1. *A warm up* serves to prepare the body and mind for the upcoming challenge. The goal is to raise body temperature and loosen muscles to obtain the greatest range of motion and flexibility. It can essentially 'teach' the body the moves that make up the HIIT

workout by practicing correct form and posture.

2. ***The performance training*** or work interval addresses power, speed, agility and sport-specific skills. Sprinters focus on the legs, weight lifters focus on the arms, shoulders and back, football players focus on the core, legs and arms, etc.

3. ***The recovery phase*** returns the body to its resting state and should include stretches and mild cardio such as brisk walking.

In fact, the inclusion of a wider range of activities helps to avoid injury since there are many muscles involved in most activities that aren't specifically related to the actual activity. For example, weight lifters need strong legs, hips and back in addition to arms and shoulders.

How HIIT Cardio Boosts Weight Training Success

When you use HIIT as a cardio workout, you can **add weight training after roughly one hour** to enhance mitochondrial biogenesis by turning on specific metabolic pathways. In this way, you ultimately increase your ability to create glycogen which is used during anaerobic activity such as extreme weight lifting. Ideally, you should perform high rep instead of high weight strength training for HIIT endurance or cardio workouts and save the heavy weight for non-HIIT workout days.

For maximum muscle growth, HIIT workouts can occur in four week cycles where you add HIIT to your training for 4 weeks then don't include it for 4 weeks. During the 'off' weeks, concentrate on muscle development and growth which will be supported by the metabolic groundwork laid by the HIIT sessions.

A Word About Nutritional Supplements

There is a lot of debate about the need for and effectiveness of nutritional supplements. The common belief is that the diet should provide everything the body requires for daily function and that supplements are a waste of money.

While that may be true in general, for athletes and hard core body builders, the **use of supplements can actually enhance the hormonal environment and stimulate the production of insulin and growth hormones for increased muscle growth.**

For overall health, fish oil and multi-vitamins with good concentrations of B, C and D provide a wide range of nutrients to support the heart, cardio vascular health and overall cellular functioning. The real issue is improving the overall diet to include as many natural sources of healthy components as possible.

Other **supplements that seem to benefit muscle building** and are commonly used include:

Beta Alanine

Beta-Ecdysterone

Branch-Chain Amino Acids (BCAA)

Caffeine

Carnitine

Casein

Conjugated Linoleic Acid

Creatine

Glutamine

High molecular weight Carbs

Lucine

Nitric Oxide Boosters

Whey protein

ZMA (zinc, magnesium aspartate, vitamin B6)

Some studies show success with many of these elements while others seem to question their effectiveness but that is beyond the scope of this text.

From my personal experience, BCAAs, Glutamine and Creatine are the ones which seemed to have the best impact on performance.

CHAPTER 9 – SAMPLE EXERCISES AND HOW TO PERFORM THEM

Bodyweight Lunge

Begin standing up straight with your feet shoulder width apart and your hands clasped loosely behind your head. Keep your left foot planted flat and step forward with your right foot in a long enough stride so that your right thigh will be parallel to the floor and your shin will be straight up and down. Return to the standing position and switch legs.

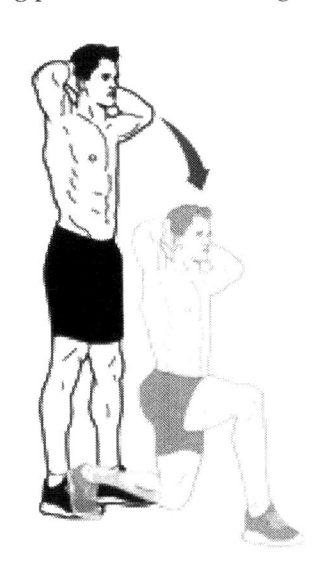

Burpee

Stand up straight with your arms at your sides and feet hip width apart. Bend your knees, allowing them to part to the side, and drop your hips as you place your hands on the ground, then kick your feet out behind you, completely dropping to the ground. Straighten your arms, arch your back and snap your feet forward while pushing yourself off the ground back into standing position.

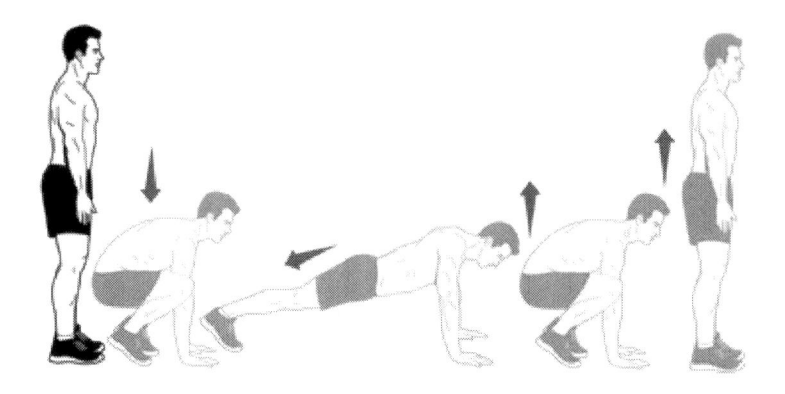

This should be a fluid, continuous movement done as quickly as possible while maintaining good form.

To make this more challenging, wear a weighted vest.

Crunch

Lie on your back, your arms crossed across your chest, with your knees bent about 60 degrees. Keep your feet flat on the floor and raise your upper body to form a 'C' while inhaling. Hold the crunch and exhale as you slowly move back to the starting position. Do not swing your arms – just use your abs to raise your torso.

HIIT

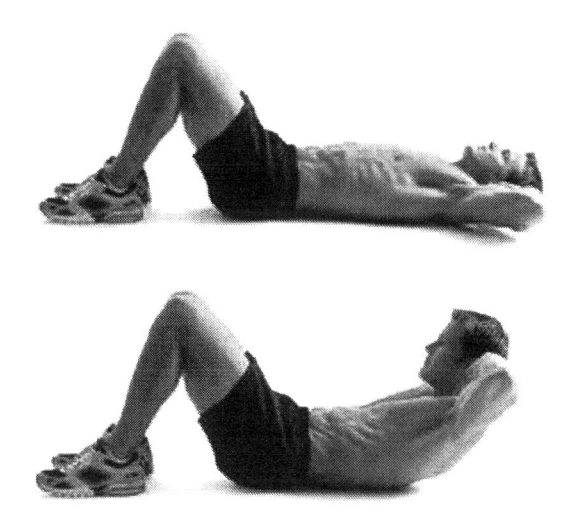

To ease the strain on your lower back, perform crunches on a Swiss ball.

For more of a challenge, hold a weight in your hands.

Heavy Ropes

In addition to climbing ropes, there are many other activities that make use of ropes for targeting a variety of muscles at different levels of intensity.

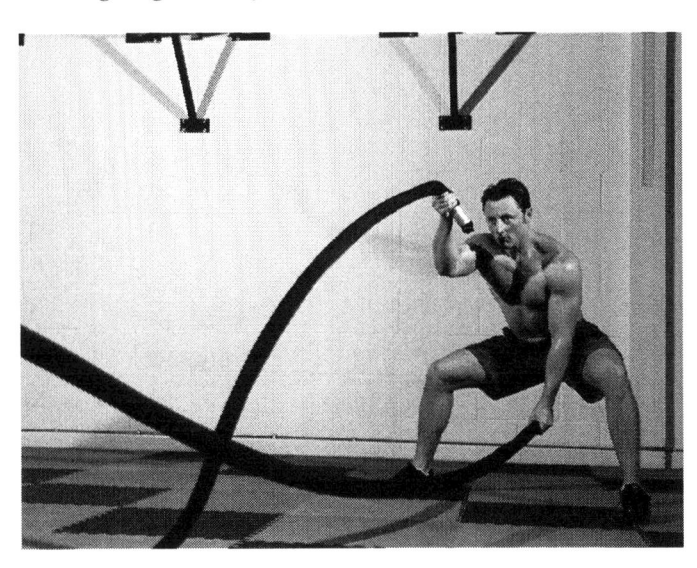

Jump Rope

A good old favorite from the playground, jumping rope is a terrific exercise that can be speed up or slowed down to suit your needs.

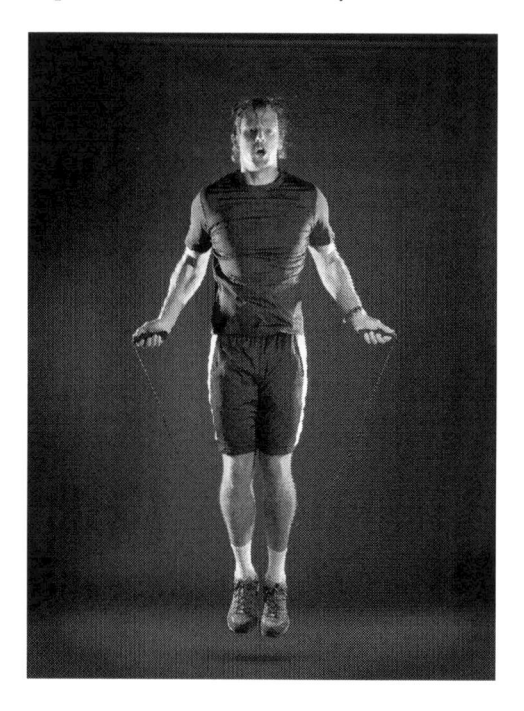

Make the activity more difficult by jumping on one foot at a time or by jumping as high as possible.

Kettlebell Swing

Stand up straight with feet slightly wider than should width and toes pointing slightly outward. Unlock your hips and bend your knees keeping your weight to the back (as if you are going to sit on a chair). With both hands, grasp the kettlebell without stretching arms – the kettlebell should only be about one foot in front of your feet. Swing the kettlebell back between your legs as you stand and use the momentum of your hips to continue swinging the kettlebell back and forth.

HIIT

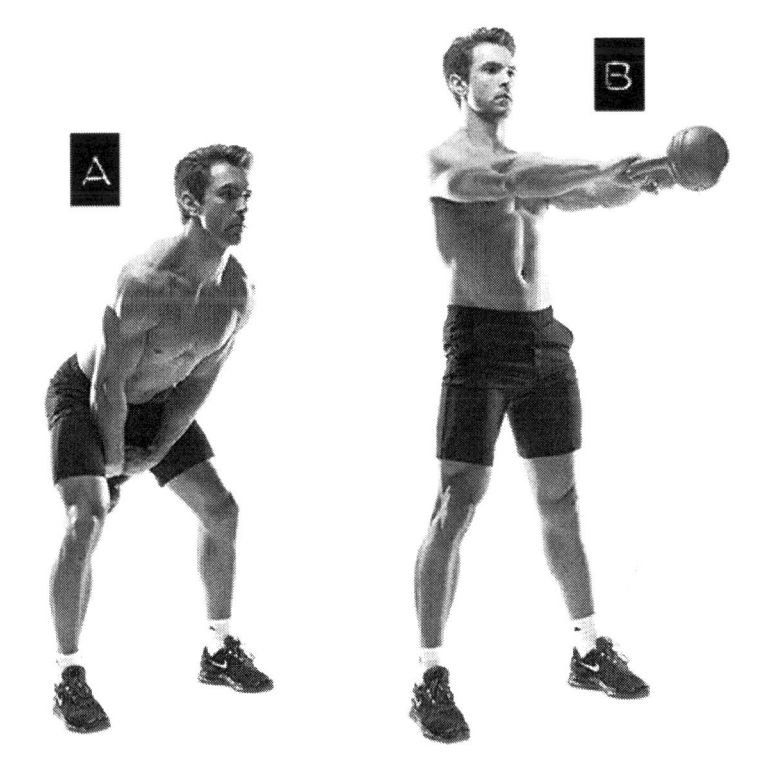

Do not tuck your chin or hyperextend your neck.

Use power breathing during the kettlebell swing.

Note that there are plenty other kettlebell exercises which are perfect for HIIT sessions – kettlebell swing is just one of them.

Mountain Climber

Begin with a push up position with your hands placed a bit below and slightly than your shoulders. Alternate bringing your knees up to your chest and stretching them out again, almost like running in place. Keep your back as straight as possible without letting your hips drop. For more of a challenge, bend your arms slightly.

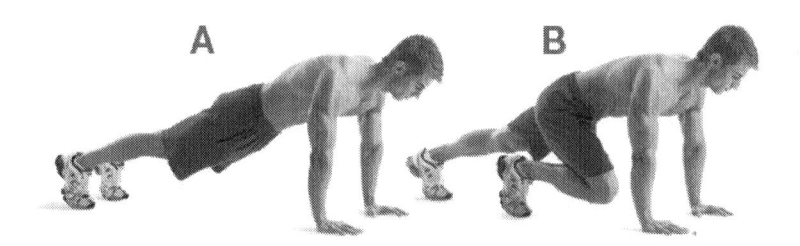

Plank

Begin as in a push up but place your elbows and forearms on the floor, hands extended straight in front. Raise your body keeping your back straight and hold this position for at least 30 seconds while bracing your core and breathing deeply.

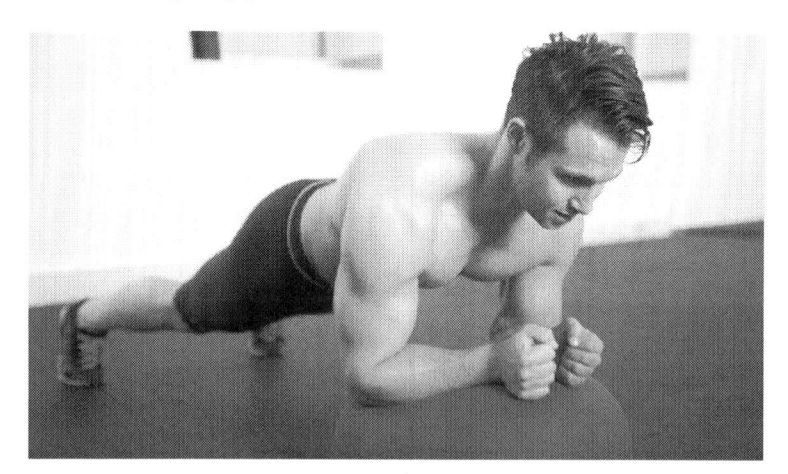

To make this easier, rest on your knees with your ankles crossed in the air.

To make this more challenging, rest your weight on your palms out in front of your head with your arms extended.

Side Plank

Lie down on your side with your feet together (one on top of the other) and raise yourself up on the bottom elbow. Place the upper hand on the raised hip and keep your core tight while breathing deeply. Maintain a straight line from your ankles to your shoulders. Hold the position, lower yourself and switch sides.

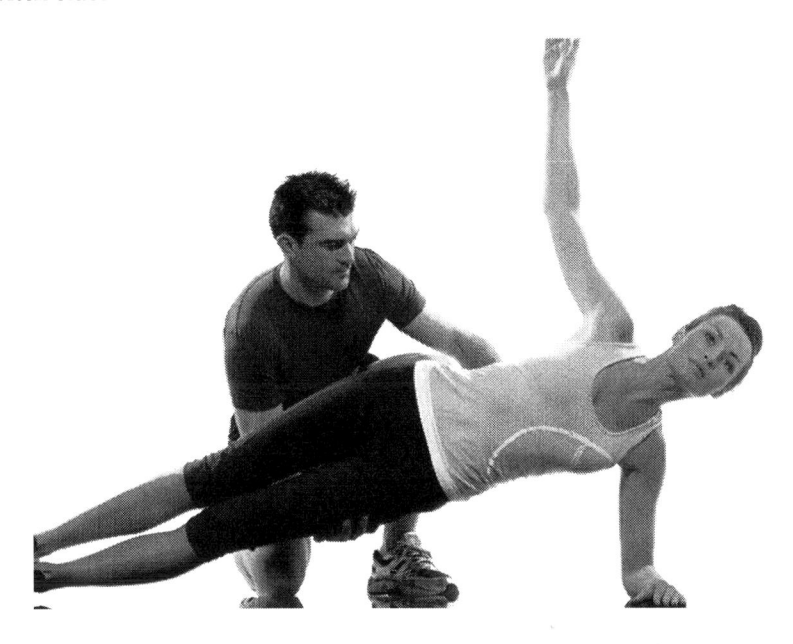

To make this easier, rest on your knees with your legs bent at 90degrees, feet behind you.

For added difficulty, raise your top leg and swing it back and forth.

Another challenging variation is to roll forward into a regular plank maintaining straight lines and a tight core.

Push Up

Begin lying on the floor (on a mat), face down. Place your hands flat on the ground, shoulder width apart, and your toes against the floor. Push up so that your arms are almost fully extended, keeping your back straight. Keep your elbows in close to your body – not pointing away. The slower the movement, the more intense the workout!

HAND PLACEMENT

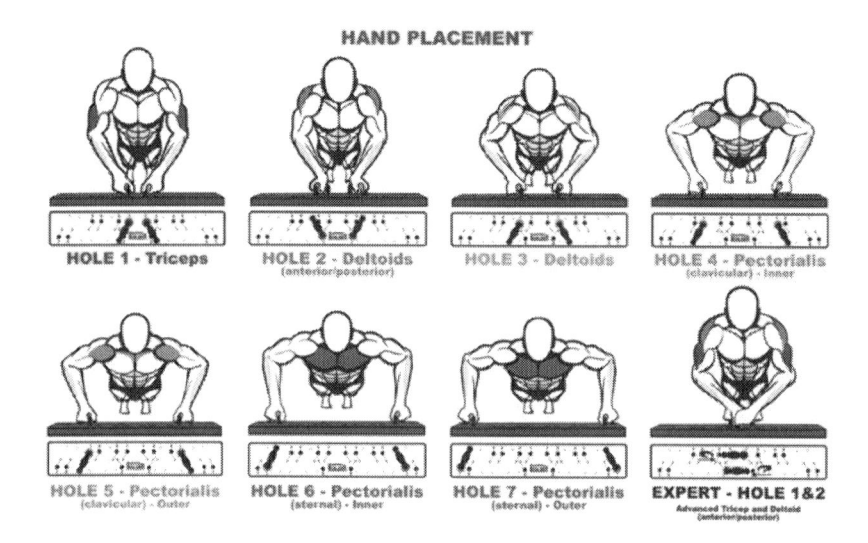

HOLE 1 - Triceps
HOLE 2 - Deltoids (anterior/posterior)
HOLE 3 - Deltoids
HOLE 4 - Pectorialis (clavicular) - Inner
HOLE 5 - Pectorialis (clavicular) - Outer
HOLE 6 - Pectorialis (sternal) - Inner
HOLE 7 - Pectorialis (sternal) - Outer
EXPERT - HOLE 1 & 2 Advanced Triceps and Deltoid (anterior/posterior)

Inhale as you bend your arms to lower your body, nearly touching your chest to the floor. Exhale as you push up off of the ground.

To make this easier, you can rest on your knees instead of your toes or perform the motion in a standing position, leaning against a wall.

To make this more challenging, elevate your feet on a platform or push up with enough force to be able to clap your hands together before lowering yourself.

Squats

With your hands wide on the barbell resting on your traps (not your neck), inhale and bend your knees as if you are going to sit on a chair. Arch your back slightly and keep your chest forward. When you reach the 'seated' position, exhale and push off from your heels to straighten your legs to return to a standing position. Instead of a barbell, you can use a dumbbell hanging at your side in each hand.

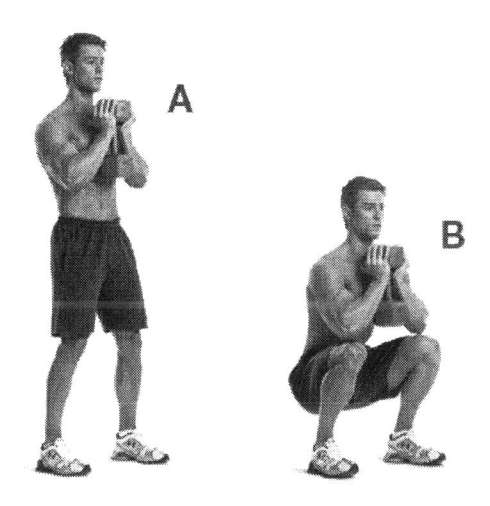

Bicep Curls

Using dumbbells or machines, working both arms together or one at a time, toning the biceps is easy and the effort can readily be tailored to anyone's ability. Standing with feet hip-width apart, core engaged, hold dumbbells in front of thighs. Curl the weights up while keeping the elbows stationary. Slowly lower the weights until the arms are almost fully extended. Slow, smooth motions provide the best results.

Bicep curls can be used for recovery activities as well as for HIIT workout.

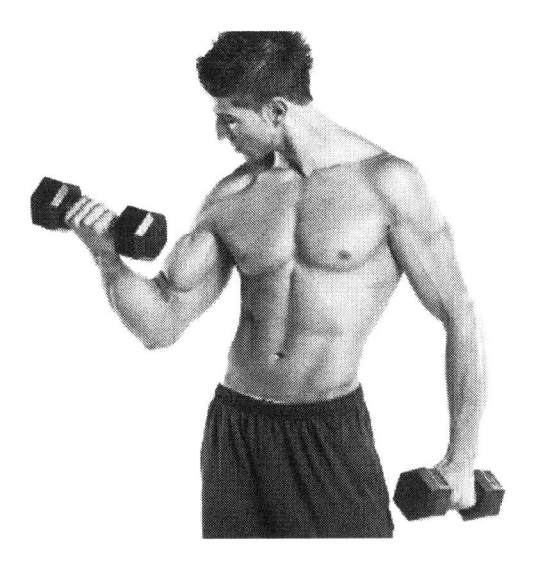

Tricep Dips

Tricep dips are easy to do with your own body weight or machines at a gym. Stand with your back to a sturdy chair or bench, placing your hands flat on the bench slightly closer together than shoulder width, knuckles facing forward. Lower your body, bending at the elbow, exhaling as you bend, until your knees are at a 90° angle. Elbows should remain in close and not point outwards. Straighten your arms slowly, inhaling on the way up.

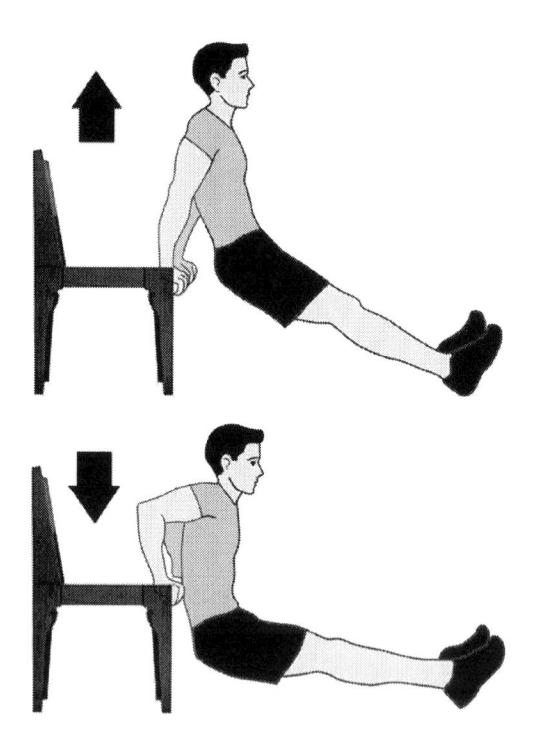

Similar as bicep curls, tricep dips can be perfectly used as part of the recovery activities if not as an actual HIIT component.

Exercise Options for HIIT Workouts

Sample HIIT Exercises for Interval Training

	Beginner	Moderate	Advanced
Walk/run	Power walk or light jog	Sprint run w/ high knees	Explosive sprint runs
Burpees	Simple Burpee	Full Burpee	Jump Burpee
Jumping Jacks	Side Step Taps	Jumping Jacks	Star Jumps from crouch
Lunges	Static Lunges w/ support	Walk lunges	Jump lunges
Press Ups	Incline press ups	Full press ups	Clap or one leg press ups
Squats	Plain squats	Medicine ball squats	Deep squats w/ jumps

20 Minute HIIT Workout

Perform each exercise for 45 seconds at full intensity followed by 90 seconds of recovery level activity.

(Warm up and cool down for 5 minutes!)

1. Push ups
2. Squats
3. Planks
4. Jump Squats
5. Crunches
6. Mountain Climbers
7. Lunges
8. Burpees
9. Triceps Dips
10. High Knees

HIIT Lower Body Workout (Bodyweight with Treadmill)

1. **Treadmill** - Warm up at 0 incline, speed at 3.5 for 5 minutes
2. **Walking lunges** for 1 minute
3. **Treadmill** - Incline at 7, speed at 3.8 for 2 minutes
4. **Standing Squats** for 1 minute
5. **Treadmill** - Incline at 9, speed at 3.6 for 2 minutes
6. **Jumping Lunges** for 1 minute
7. **Treadmill** - Incline at 11, speed at 3.4 for 2 minutes
8. **Jumping Squats** for 1 minute
9. **Treadmill** - Incline at 13, speed at 3.2 for 2 minutes
10. **Jumping Squats** with **Jumping Lunges** for 1 minute
11. **Treadmill** - Incline at 15, speed at 3.0 for 2 minutes
12. **Treadmill** - Cool down at 0 incline, speed at 3.5 for 5 minutes

HIIT Upper Body Workout

Warm up with easy cardio for 5 minutes.

Then do 5 minutes of **HIIT cardio** – 30 seconds intense, 30 seconds recovery.

Alternate 1 minute of each of the following exercises with 1 minute of stretching and then finish off with 5 minutes of easy cardio.

- V-sits

- Triceps push-ups

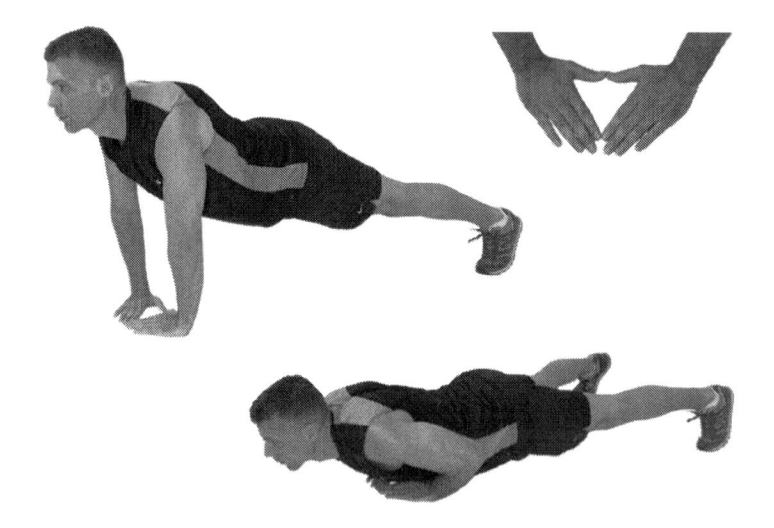

- Sit ups

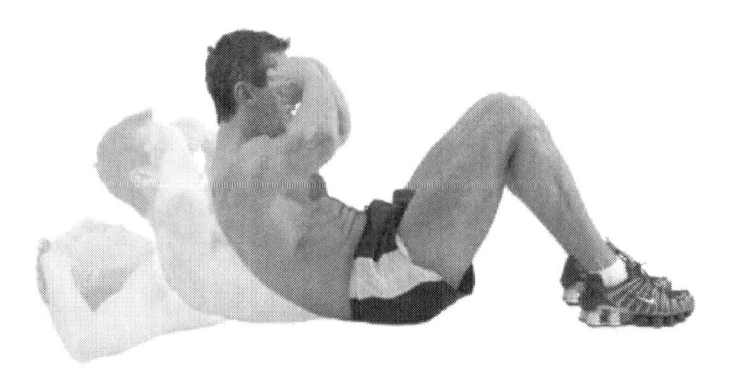

- Mountain Climbers
- Push-ups
- Bicycles
- Triceps dips
- Plank

7-Minute HIIT Workout

Perform these exercises allowing 30 seconds for each at about 80% of maximum effort. Allow 10 seconds rest between exercises. Don't forget to warm up and cool down.

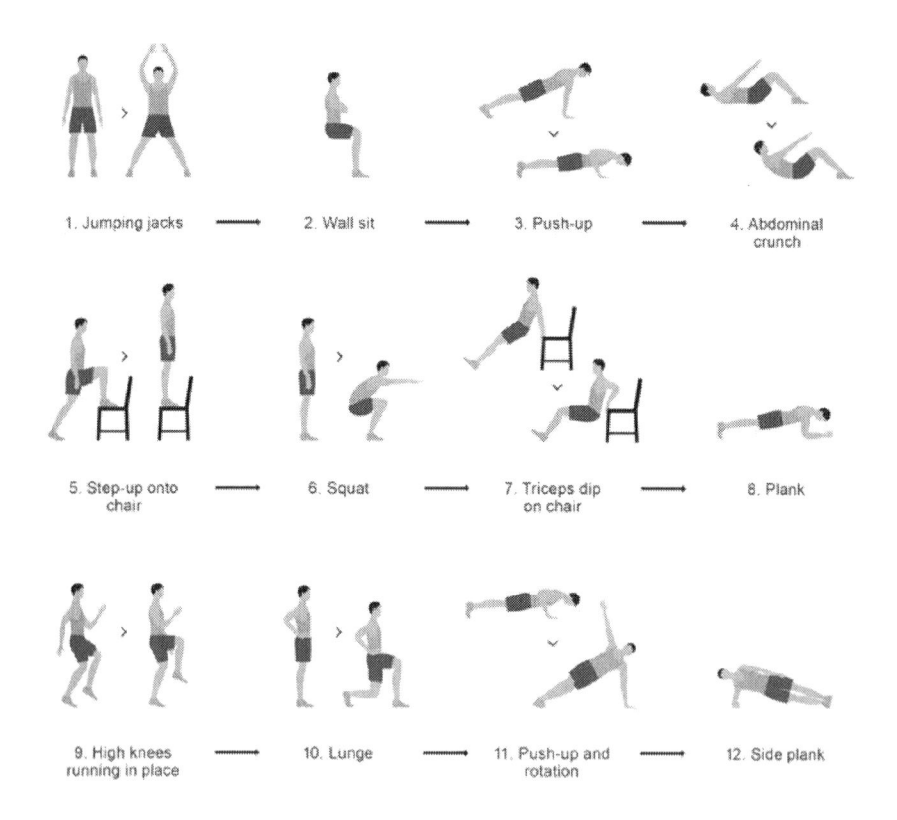

1. Jumping jacks
2. Wall sit
3. Push-up
4. Abdominal crunch
5. Step-up onto chair
6. Squat
7. Triceps dip on chair
8. Plank
9. High knees running in place
10. Lunge
11. Push-up and rotation
12. Side plank

In these 12 exercises deploying only body weight, a chair and a wall, it fulfills the latest mandates for high-intensity effort, which essentially combines a long run and a visit to the gym into about seven minutes of steady discomfort — all of it based on science!

CHAPTER 10 - FAQ

What is HIIT?

HIIT or High Intensity Interval Training is an approach to exercise that is based on alternating short intervals of high intensity activity with intervals of moderate activity for as little as 4 minutes or as much as 30 minutes.

Is HIIT approved by professionals?

HIIT is the result of experience and research in the field of sports physiology. Many studies support the benefits of HIIT in terms of physical fitness and overall health.

Who can perform HIIT workouts?

Virtually anyone can perform HIIT workouts because it is based on an individual's maximum effort and not a specific number of repetitions, distance to be covered or weight to move. It is adaptable for people of all ages and physical abilities.

How can I start a HIIT program?

Any activity can be used in a HIIT program- it is just a matter of intensity and timing. Running, calisthenics, swimming, circuit training- anything you do that you can work at near maximum heart rate for up to 2 minutes then drop back to moderate heart rate for 'recovery' can be a HIIT activity.

Is a HIIT program expensive?

HIIT can be performed at home or in a gym with just body weight or minimal equipment. Almost any activity can be adapted to become a HIIT workout.

Is weight training a HIIT activity?

Weight training can be a HIIT activity but it requires dropping back to roughly 50% of your usual weights. In order to maintain maximum heart rate for the required length of time, you have to work at a lower weight. Another consideration is the energy burn and stress to the CNS that occurs in a HIIT workout. Such intensity may leave your body without the resources it needs to follow up with your regular weight training program.

What is VO2max?

VO2max refers to the maximum amount of oxygen a person can utilize during intense exercise and is the measure of an athlete's cardiovascular fitness and level of endurance.

What is Afterburn?

EPOC -'excess post-exercise oxygen consumption'- is the body's way of returning the metabolism to 'normal' after heavy exercise. This is because the body continues to consume oxygen to supply cellular energy needs that have been depleted through intense activity such as HIIT, which is designed to maximize intensity.

What is lactate threshold?

This is the point at which the body has produced so much lactic acid during intense activity and anaerobic metabolism that it can no longer be removed efficiently. The lactic acid begins to build up in the muscles and reduces the power of contractions while leading to exhaustion.

What is ATP?

ATP (adenosine triphosphate) is a molecule which is the fuel that powers the human body. When one of the phospates is removed, the result is ADP which is then re-powered in the mitochondria to function again as ATP.

What are mitochondria?

Within each cell, mitochondria produce energy for cellular function and are an active element of metabolism. They also contribute to the building of certain elements of blood, store calcium ions needed for nerve function and help detoxify ammonia in the liver.

What is glycogen?

Glycogen is the way glucose (blood sugar) is stored in the body for later use. It is produced in the liver but stored in the muscles and fat cells where it can be retrieved for conversion to blood glucose for cellular function.

What is overtraining?

Overtraining is simply pushing the body too hard and not allowing enough time for muscle recovery and the stabilization of body chemicals. Symptoms include decreased performance, stiffness and soreness, headaches and an overall lack of energy.

What are the best sources of protein for fitness?

Natural chicken and fish (as opposed to grain fed or farmed), Greek yogurt, shellfish, eggs, beans and soy are considered to be the healthiest sources of protein along with lean grass fed beef, pork tenderloin, milk and cheese.

Is there such a thing as 'too much protein'?

While adequate protein is necessary for muscle growth and function, too much protein can lead to kidney problems (including kidney stones), the leeching of calcium from the bones, reduced ketosis (elevation of pH in the blood when glycogen stores are depleted) and gout.

What are 'good' and 'bad' carbohydrates?

'Good' carbs don't cause spikes in blood sugar because they are more complex and require more to break them down. These include whole grains, fruits, vegetables, beans and skim milk products. 'Bad' carbs are processed sweets but also white bread (and other 'white' flour products), white rice and snacks such as potato chips and pretzels.

What are the proper percentages of foods for fitness?

10% fat from unflavored and unsweetened nuts and nut butters, olives, avocados. 25% lean protein (see sources above). 30% from fiber carbs (not sugar carbs). 35% from vegetables and fruits (raw is best). And don't forget the healthy herbs, spices, lemon juice and vinegar instead of salt and sauces!

How do I know if I am drinking enough water?

With as little as a 2% loss of fluids, the body can begin to show signs of dehydration such as dry skin, dry mouth, thirst, fatigue or weakness, chills and head rushes. More significant dehydration (5%) results in increased heart rate, respiration and temperature, decreased sweating, muscle cramps or tingling of the limbs, headaches and nausea. Severe dehydration (10% reduction in bodily fluid) can result in vomiting, muscle spasms, seizures, unconsciousness and death.

Is there any benefit to caffeine as a supplement?

Caffeine supplements provide a quick burst of energy and mental focus that may last about an hour. That is certainly within the scope of a HIIT workout. Caffeine intake (supplements of beverages) should be moderate in preparation for extensive workouts, especially those that deplete the body's store of liquid. Caffeine is a diuretic and forces water and other fluids out of the body so adequate hydration may be hampered.

How can I get rid of my …….?

There is really no way to target a specific area for weight loss but the overall reduction of body fat and the toning of specific areas through selected HIIT activities will make a big difference.

Why do I need to warm up before exercise?

There are numerous reasons to warm up: to increase the temperature of the body, muscles and blood, to dilate the blood vessels, to loosen the muscles and improve range of motion, to increase the production of certain hormones responsible for energy production and to prepare yourself mentally for the activity to follow.

When should I stretch?

Stretching should follow activity so that the muscles have warmed up. There is always a risk of injuring a cold muscle if it is pulled too far. During a warm up session, begin with light aerobics to get the blood flowing then move to stretching. Stretching is also helpful after a workout to let the muscles and heart rate gradually return to normal so that they don't stiffen up or so that blood can continue to flow smoothly and not get 'trapped' in suddenly inactive muscles.

Why is the core so important?

This group of muscles is responsible for stabilizing the body (maintaining balance), protecting the spine and spinal cord and providing strong support for the limbs so they work well. They are made up of layers of muscles – externals, internals, front, sides and back.

How do I pick the right HIIT intervals?

The 'right' HIIT intervals are the ones that you can achieve consistently with the maximum effort. If you don't work hard enough, you won't see the best results so the interval has to be short enough that you can give it 95% but long enough that it isn't easy. After the rest intervals, you should be able to give it almost the same intensity until you just can't give any more. Maximum effort means maximum exhaustion when the workout is over. That's why HIIT workouts don't usually last more than 20 – 30 minutes.

How is maximum heart rate determined?

As a general rule, HR max is determined by subtracting your age from 220. During exercise, you should typically work between 50 and 85% of your maximum heart rate but HIIT workouts will keep you at the higher end. It is important to note that some medications affect the heart rate so the target zone needs to be adjusted. As always, before beginning an exercise program, consult with your health care professional.

How can the intensity of HIIT exercise be increased if it seems too easy?

The easiest way to increase the intensity of any exercise is to add weights – either a weighted vest, a flat plate or dumbbells. With many bodyweight exercises, changing elevations can also increase the intensity such as working on a Swiss ball or Bosu ball or raising your feet for push-ups. Adding a jump during standing exercises or a clap during push-ups makes them more difficult as does performing them with just one leg or arm.

CONCLUSION

Fit and fantastic – that is the result of participating in HIIT workouts. HIIT is a well-researched method of achieving physical fitness and optimal body functioning while reducing weight and improving cardiovascular health and flexibility.

HIIT offers many benefits to both the beginner and advanced athlete through the options for timing workout and recovery intervals and the numerous choices of activities for all aspects of strength and conditioning. With adjustments in diet and attention to proper hydration and adequate recovery and rest, virtually anyone can improve their overall fitness in as little as 2 weeks or just 20 minutes a day.

Healthy living is a habit that needs to be nurtured and encouraged. By adding HIIT workouts to your weekly routine, you can quickly address exercise and leave more time to other pursuits. HIIT activities can be taken from your favorite competitive or individual sports and leisure pastimes such as dancing, skiing or hiking, no matter what time of year, indoors or outdoors.

Changing your eating habits is always a challenge but the demands of HIIT naturally lead you to making better dietary choices. With a little common sense and guidance, it is fairly simple to avoid the 'bad' foods that pack on the pounds and switch to those that enhance your metabolism and digestion.

Weight lifting, body building, endurance and cardio HIIT routines provide nearly countless opportunities to focus on particular parts of the body or create a well-rounded routine that addresses all the major muscle groups. Toning, shaping and creating a six pack have never been easier!

HIIT activities can just as easily be done at home as in a gym with body weight activities or minimal equipment. Circuit training enthusiasts can adapt any piece of gym equipment as well as weights to HIIT routines and different cardio choices can be made for any day of the week.

With so many possibilities, there is certainly some activity that you can adapt into a HIIT workout plan. Take what you already know and go from there or try some of the many suggestions throughout this book – it is just a matter of alternating hard work with moderate exercise to spark the metabolism and promote muscle growth and overall fitness.

For a terrific challenge that promises plenty of fantastic results, HIIT workouts will take you to a fitness level you never would have believed possible!

ABOUT THE AUTHOR

When John was young, he did not have much interest in sports. As a young boy, his main pursuits were reading and video games. It was not until he entered elementary school and started to be bullied that he gained a desire to start training his body. Though he was already a couple years behind the kinds that had started out in peewee soccer, football, and tennis, he quickly caught up and was pleased to find that the mental dexterity and alertness that reading and video games had developed improved his performance on the field.

By the time he entered high school, he was one of the best players on the team. That is when John's coach pulled him aside and asked him to rev up his training regimen. John was already training as hard as he could, he thought, but it was clear that he was not doing enough. Instead of killing himself in the gym every day after school, John started researching different training methods, and ran across something called high intensity training. It wasn't just about training harder, it was about training smarter–doing the right exercises at the right time, training the entire body and the mind to withstand more.

By the time he was finished with college, he was learning as much as he could about how to improve the body's performance and how to efficiently exercise to get the results he was looking for, from using kettlebells, to just pumping iron.

It was in college that he started body building and training with High Intensity Interval Training programs, and since that time, he has dedicated his life to learning as much as he possible can about different kinds of exercise.

When he came across HIIT training, he knew he had stumbled onto something completely new and incredible. It was a program that could tone the body and shape the mind, teaching your body how to burn fat efficiently, especially when paired with the right diet. Most of all, it was far more enjoyable for most people, even for people who hated exercising. When he realized this, it became his life's mission to bring High Intensity Interval Training to the world, to a whole new audience of people who could benefit not only from the workouts, but from the improved mindset that HIIT training produced.

With the hatred and dread of working out removed from the picture, he found that his personal training clients were much more willing to put in the work to achieve the bodies they desired. HIIT soon became the forefront of his training, working with everyday people and with athletes, all of whom have benefitted from his expertise in this program. Years of training with HIIT and sharing his knowledge have made John one of the foremost experts on this incredible workout regimen.

Printed in Great Britain
by Amazon